THE **COMPLETE GUIDE** TO

Jon Ackland

ENDURANCE TRAINING

3rd edition

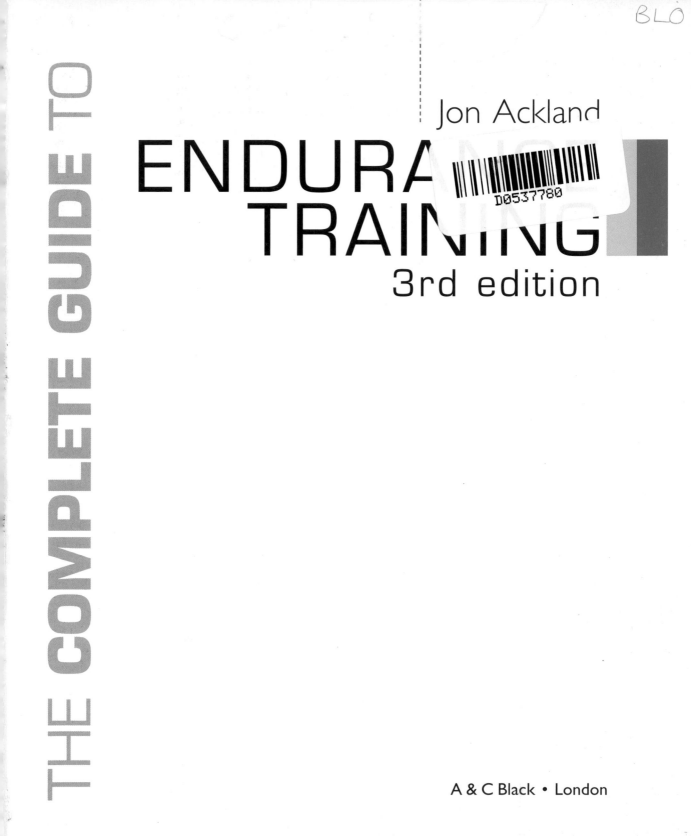

A & C Black • London

Note

Whilst every effort has been made to ensure that the content of this book is as technically accurate and as sound as possible, neither the editors nor the publisher can accept responsibility for any injury or loss sustained as a result of the use of this material.

Jon Ackland is the director of Performance Lab Intl., a specialist training programme prescription and assessment facility for athletes. Training Programmes are regularly produced for athletes all over the world competing or completing successfully in a wide range of events. Information for beginners, recreational, advanced and elite athletes is available by contacting them:

Web Site : www.performancelab.co.nz
Email: info@performancelab.co.nz
Phone: +64 9 480 1422
Fax: +64 9 480 1423
Address: P.O. Box 34 174
Birkenhead
North Shore City,
New Zealand

Published by A & C Black Publishers Ltd
38 Soho Square, London W1D 3HB

Third edition 2007

First edition 1999
Second edition 2003

Previously published as
The Power to Perform

Published by special arrangement with
Reed Books, a division of Reed Publishing (NZ) Ltd
39 Raewene Rd, Birkenhead, Auckland

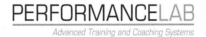

Copyright © 2007, 2003, 1999 Jon Ackland and Brett Reid

ISBN 9780713679038

A CIP catalogue record for this book is available from the British Library.

Thank you to Anita Bean for her contribution to Chapter 12, 'Sports Nutrition, Race Rehydration and Refuelling'.

I would like to thank the team at A&C Black for their patience.
Producing this new edition was no easy task!

Illustrations © Dave Saunders

This book is produced using paper that is made from wood grown in managed, sustainable forests. It is natural, renewable and recyclable. The logging and manufacturing processes conform to the environmental regulations of the country of origin.

Typeset in 10.5 on 12.5pt Baskerville BE Regular by Palimpsest Book Production Ltd, Grangemouth, Stirlingshire

Printed and bound in Italy by Rotolito

ACKNOWLEDGEMENTS

This book is dedicated

- To my Mum and Dad (Maureen and Jim) and my sister (Jill) who have always supported and encouraged me. Thanks for all you have done for me throughout my life.

- To my wonderful partner, Kerri McMaster, who supported me tremendously in the writing of this book, and whose patience, wisdom and encouragement get me through life. A special thank you to Anne McMaster, whose constant support and care have helped me beyond words in the last few years.

- To my mentors and heroes, who unselfishly taught me what I needed to know about exercise and training. They are Gary Regtien, Jim Blair and the late Sam Johnson. The world would be a better place with a few more of you guys. Thanks for everything.

- Finally, to Arthur Lydiard, whose ideas revolutionised endurance training.

CONTENTS

Foreword   v
Preface   vi

PART ONE Training Basics   1

1 Understanding Your Training   2
2 The Principles of Training   10
3 Recovery, Training Intensities and Heart Rates   27
4 Training Subphases   48
5 Manipulation of Training Principles   65
6 Fundamentals that Aid Training and Performance   100

PART TWO Taking It to the Next Level   131

7   How to Write Your Own Programme   132
8   Analysing Your Training   164
9   Preparing for Race Day   167
10 The Coach   177
11 The Environment – Altitude, Heat, Cold and Travel   180
12 Sports Nutrition, Race Rehydration and Refuelling   195

PART THREE Specific Sample Programmes   209

13 Triathlon Training Programmes   224
14 Duathlon Training Programmes   246
15 Multi-sport Training Programmes   252
16 Rowing and Kayaking Training Programmes   260
17 Road Cycling Training Programmes   264
18 Mountain Biking Training Programmes   276
19 Distance Running Training Programmes   280

Appendix   292
Bibliography   294
Recommended Reading   296
Index   297

FOREWORD

It is very seldom that a book can simultaneously meet the learning and practical application needs of both athlete and coach. *The Complete Guide to Endurance Training* is one such book and has established the benchmark against which all training guides will be measured in future.

The guide is written in such a style that the diverse and complex issues of developing and preparing athletes for endurance sports are made perfectly understandable: training theory and practical programme design are clearly and concisely explained. Jon Ackland really knows the subject because he has been there.

Most impressive of all is the thorough attention to practical detail as the reader is guided through the steps of planning programmes that are designed to meet the needs of the athlete or the coach at their own level of development.

The Complete Guide to Endurance Training is essential reading for anyone involved in triathlon, Ironman, duathlon, distance running, cycle racing, mountain biking, rowing and all other forms of endurance activity.

Frank W. Dick O.B.E.
President, European Athletics Coaches Association
Author, *Sports Training Principles*

PREFACE

I am currently sitting at my desk in Valencia. The team I am working with is called Emirates Team New Zealand. They are an America's Cup yachting syndicate and we are in the semi-finals. We have spent 3 years preparing for this and things are going well so far.

The interesting thing is that despite all the money, technology, testing and race preparation it is amazing how much team unity, mental toughness, momentum and belief play a part in winning.

When I first wrote *The Complete Guide to Endurance Training* I thought it was all about the training you did. Were 3 reps of a particular type of training better than 4? While this is still important, what I have learnt in the last few years is how much other areas of performance contribute to the final result.

The first is going back to basics. It becomes increasingly obvious that spending 20% of your time thinking and planning and 80% of your time training is much more powerful than 1% of your time thinking and 99% of your time training. If you have a blurry idea of what you need to achieve, your training will be blurry and the result will be blurry. Make sure you spend enough time setting your goals and then setting up clear steps to achieving them. Pretty obvious stuff, huh? Not many athletes do this well!

Other simple things become clearer. The better you understand what you are getting into the better your plan, the better your preparation and the better a job you do in the race. Simple stuff but we often don't spend enough time on the basics.

Secondly, there are two parts to performance. These are preparation: the training you do, and execution: the strategy and ability to execute your preparation in a race. Now the interesting thing here is that you can do fantastic preparation but on the day you might use 100% of that preparation or you might only use 30% of it. It does not automatically follow that if you've done the training you're going to get it right. Anyone who has had to sell or present anything will testify to this. So you must have a preparation plan (training programme) but you should also have a very clear race strategy. In fact to some degree the race strategy is more important than the training plan, as to some extent your strategy drives what you prepare for.

Your head has a huge influence on how you perform. It effects how stable you are as you train – not getting caught up in racing your training partners and pushing your training too hard or too early. It affects how you handle the pressure and what you focus on in competition, which has a significant effect on the final result. It is interesting that most athletes overtrain their bodies but undertrain their minds. It fact many never train their minds at all.

It is with this in mind that I have added the new additions to the text – it needed to be complete! Lastly, it brings up the concept of 'complete performance' and striving to better yourself in all of the aspects that make up a champion; and this applies to any athlete of any level. You can improve significantly if you choose to apply yourself and work at being better and draw an enormous amount of fulfillment and satisfaction breaking new boundaries and reaching new levels of ability, control and understanding.

Jon Ackland
May, 2007

PART **ONE**

TRAINING BASICS

UNDERSTANDING YOUR TRAINING

Understand, save time, maximise returns

Healthy or sick, rich or poor, famous or anonymous, we are all Time's obedient servants; each of us is obliged to admit that there are only so many hours in the day. Yet how many of us value time in the same way that we value money? Or diamonds? Or gold? Time is money, they say. But it's not. It's far more valuable, especially to an endurance athlete. Many hours of training have to be fitted in around education, work, family and the daily chores that make up a life. It is absolutely crucial, therefore, that training is as efficient as possible, with little or no wastage of time and/or effort.

For instance, ask yourself this question: is all my training and effort giving me the best possible result in terms of fun, health and racing performance? I believe few athletes can honestly answer that question with an emphatic Yes! To avoid the twin demons of wasted time and wasted effort, it is necessary to design a training programme that is specific to your needs (competitive or otherwise). But before you do this you must know where you are going. What are your goals for the year? How are you going to achieve them? What was the aim of last month's training? Did you achieve it? What training have you got planned for tomorrow? Why? Until you can answer these questions, and many more like them, it is unlikely you will achieve the success you deserve from your efforts.

The key to realising your racing potential is understanding your training. In New Zealand we have a phrase, 'All the gears and no ideas'. Too many athletes could put this on their gravestone; much better to live under the banner 'Knowledge is power', for once you understand how to train effectively, not only will you improve, but you will also enjoy yourself far more in the process. The most common misconception held by endurance athletes is that more is better. Too often this translates to 'garbage in, garbage out'. Generally, most endurance athletes need to train less – but more efficiently. For example, planning and analysing your training for ten minutes a week may be far more effective than doing another two hours of hard work. It's certainly more fun!

Thought should also be given to technique and equipment. Improvements in both these areas may yield far better results than simply doing more miles 'in the wrong position on the wrong bike'. A good example of this approach is the overweight athlete on an ultra-lightweight racing bike with aero helmet, disk wheels and a bad back, which forces him/her to ride in an upright position! A structured programme would not only bring better results and prevent injuries, but it might save the athlete several thousand pounds in equipment. Of course, good equipment can help you get the best out of yourself, and might even make training more enjoyable, but it's not the crucial factor. Efficient use of time and resources, that's the key.

Make a plan

The planning of each training week and month is vital if you want to achieve optimal performance. Many athletes put a lot of effort into training without carefully setting a programme that will bring improvement. After all, if you are going to dedicate considerable time and effort to your training, the least you can do is sit down and plan it! Right? Always aim to schedule 30 minutes planning time into your weekly training programme. Use this time to analyse what you have done and plan what you are going to do.

'Listen' to your body both during and after training. Did last week's speed session flatten you too much? Did you do too many miles? Let the way you feel and respond to different types of training guide you as you work out your programme. You alone will be the best judge of the type, volume and intensity of training that is best for you.

Monitor every aspect of training and note how it feels. This will give you a much better idea of how to pinpoint training errors and successes. And remember, bad performances and workouts can be just as beneficial if you learn from them. If you can continue to refine your training through analysis and planning, you will waste less time and perform far better.

As one top competitor has said, 'Champion athletes have two types of days – good days, and days where they learn something'. In other words, Train Smart!

Basic training concepts

1 Specificity

You race how you train. If you train slowly, you race slowly. If you train over short distances, you will only be able to race short distances.

Training should simulate how you intend to race. The closer you get to race day, the stronger that simulation should be. Only by applying the principle of specificity will you be able to prepare your body properly for racing.

2 Frequency

To improve a certain aspect of your physical ability you will need to practise that aspect repeatedly. Crash training programmes normally result in you becoming injured or overtrained. Frequency also means consistency – a little, often is much better than a lot, seldom.

3 Overload

Workouts must overload your system if they are to promote the adaptation process. By adapting to greater and greater training workloads (stress), your ability in specific aspects of performance will improve.

4 Recovery

This is crucial. Recovery fosters improvement. An athlete who doesn't recover adequately from workouts will fail to improve, for it is during recovery, not training, that the adaptation to training (growth) occurs. Remember: training plus recovery equals improvement!

5 Reversibility

Training effects are reversible. If you don't train, or train less, you will (in the long term) lose fitness and performance.

6 Flexibility

Your training plan must be able to cope with unexpected developments at work, at home and in your physical condition. You must also be able to adapt to different types of racing and racing conditions. A good training programme and athlete are flexible.

7 Adaptability

Training volumes and intensities must be increased gradually. Only then will your body adapt to the increasing demands being placed upon it. Adaptation cannot be rushed!

8 Maintenance

During the off-season you should try to maintain some of the gains you made during the last competitive season. Do this by following an easy, low-intensity programme. Make it fun.

9 Listen to your body

Always listen to your body before, and during, training. A programme designed in advance cannot take into account the way you feel on any particular day. Some days you will be too tired to do the workout on your programme. On those days ignore the programme and take it easy. You are not a machine!

10 Quality vs quantity

The correct type of training, at the right intensity, for the right duration, will bring better results than simply doing high mileage for the sake of it. Don't get sucked in by the 'more is better' school of training. Think before you train.

11 Goal setting

Set achievable, realistic goals based on where you are at right now. These goals should cover the next few weeks (short-term goals), the next twelve months (intermediate goals) and your entire sporting career (long-term goals). If you don't achieve a goal, don't get despondent. Sit down and see if you can learn something about your preparation, your racing tactics or your goal-setting strategy. Good athletes don't have good days and bad days, they have good days and learning days.

12 Trainability

Training improvements do not occur consistently over time. There will be periods when you improve a lot, and there will be times when you don't seem to be making any progress at all. Improvements tend to be greatest early on in a training programme. The cumulative fatigue that results from high mileage can make you feel like you are on a performance plateau during high mileage phases. The answer? Hang in there and be patient!

13 Warming up, warming down

Try to warm up before every workout, especially before speedwork or other high-intensity sessions. This will reduce the risk of injury and improve the quality of the workout. Warm-downs will help flush out by-products in the muscles. This promotes faster recovery and means you will be better prepared for your next workout.

14 Technique

A good technique will make you a better athlete. Take the time to refine your technique.

The components of training

By understanding and controlling the following training components, you will train and compete more effectively.

1 Intensity

Intensity is the effort or energy required for a particular form of training. The intensity of the workout must be sufficiently stressful to allow adaptation to overload to occur.

2 Duration

This is the length of time it takes to complete a workout.

3 Volume

Volume is a measure (miles/km, hours/minutes) of how much work you perform during a workout. Intensity and volume are inversely related – the more intense the workout, the lower the volume of the workout.

4 Rest periods

Rest periods are the length of time between periods of training, for example between intervals or sprints or workouts. The length of the rest period depends on the relationship between the intensity/volume of the workout and the athlete's tolerance to training.

5 Repetitions

Repetitions (reps) are the number of times a specific form of training is completed during a workout, for example 3 x 1km. Repetitions are generally associated with speedwork and shorter duration intervals. They are generally grouped into sets.

How long will it take you to be the best you can?

Generally, it will take at least two to five years to get close to your peak in a sport. Further increases can still occur after this (and probably will), but the increments of performance improvement will be smaller. When this starts happening, the only way to get better is to train smarter! Remember, too, that talent plays a large part in all endeavours; not everybody will reach the top in their chosen sport (you can thank your parents for that!). And if you are not one of these chosen few, then you need to set your sights on your own targets, personal bests and having fun.

The fun aspect cannot be emphasised enough. If you are not going to be an Olympic champion, and perhaps even if you are, try to keep your sport in perspective. In particular, don't turn it into another job! Also, don't try to hurry your rate of improvement. Champions are not made overnight, even if the media would sometimes like you to believe this is so. One athlete, after a journalist implied his success was awfully sudden, replied: 'Yeah, it's only taken me ten years to become an overnight sensation!'

Ten variables that can influence your sporting development

1 Talent (doing a sport that suits your physical and mental make-up)
2 Coaching
3 Log book use, analysis and refinement of training (very important)
4 Technique (skill acquisition)
5 Training specificity
6 Training frequency
7 Commitment and mental approach to the sport
8 Knowledge and experience in training and racing
9 Having a training programme that suits you
10 Equipment (generally one of the least important)

Table 1.1	Preparation time for specific events
Event	Preparation time (weeks)
Ironman triathlon	16–20
Mountain bike	12
Olympic/sprint triathlon	12
Cycle race 60–100km	12
Cycle race 160+km, tour	16–20
Rowing	12
Marathon	16–20
10km race	12
Multisport	12–20

Length of training build-up

Many athletes, both elite and novice, believe it only takes a few weeks to get fully fit for a race. Unfortunately, it is not that easy if you want to perform to your potential (and we usually do). If base training – the foundation of your fitness – is not done adequately, then the quality of your speedwork and racing will suffer accordingly. Having said that, starting specific training too soon can also pose a few problems, mainly to do with boredom and loss of enthusiasm. Don't get too keen too soon. Many athletes who do huge mileages during winter never make it to the startline come summer. In this respect, training is just like good comedy – timing is everything!

Assuming you already have a reasonable level of conditioning, Table 1.1 gives some approximate guidelines on how long it will take you to prepare (base, speedwork, taper) for a number of different events. Speedwork generally starts four to eight weeks before the race.

Why base, speed, peak?

Figure 1.1 shows the performance pyramids of two athletes. The training history of the athlete on the left (competitor 1) is less than that of the athlete on the right (competitor 2). This results in competitor 1 achieving a lower peak performance than competitor 2.

There is a logical and natural progression in training for a sport. The height of an athlete's performance pyramid is largely determined by his/her training history for a specific sport. The greater that history, the greater the base (training preparation). This is because an experienced athlete is better able to cope with larger base training volumes (they've done it all before) than the novice athlete. For an athlete, a big base provides a better tolerance to training, a faster recovery from training and the ability to handle more speedwork. All these factors add up to a potentially higher peak in performance, although other factors such as talent, specificity of training and so on can greatly influence just how well an athlete

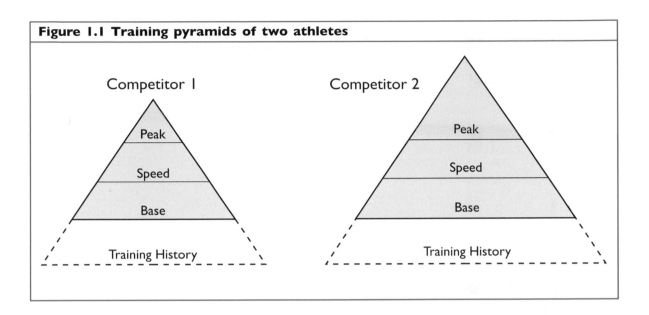

Figure 1.1 Training pyramids of two athletes

Competitor 1

Peak
Speed
Base
Training History

Competitor 2

Peak
Speed
Base
Training History

performs. Nevertheless, there is no doubt that the greater the training history, the better an athlete is likely to do.

If you haven't got time to train fully and are interested in just completing an event, table 1.2 shows the minimum number of days you should plan to train each week to finish the event comfortably.

Energy systems

The body uses two main energy systems, one of which breaks down into two further parts. These systems are:

1 The **anaerobic** energy system, which breaks down into the alactic (immediate) and lactic (non-oxidative) sub-systems.
2 The **aerobic** energy system (oxidative).

The anaerobic system

The anaerobic system is used during high-intensity exercise where energy demands exceed

Table 1.2	Minimum number of training days per week required to train for an event
Sport	Minimum no. of training days
Cycle/mountain biking	
40km (1 hr)	2
80km (2.5 hrs)	3
160km (5.5 hrs)	3–4
Tour (12 hrs over 2 days)	5–6
Triathlon sprint	3
Standard	3–4
Half-ironman	4–5
Ironman	5–6
Rowing	3-6
Running 10km	2–4
Half-marathon	4–5
Marathon	5–6

aerobic metabolism. In other words, this system is used when you are exercising without oxygen, for example in sprinting.

The *anaerobic alactic* system is used during very high-intensity exercise (maximum effort for under ten to 20 seconds) and supplies immediate energy. It does not require oxygen to function (anaerobic) and no lactic acid is produced (alactic).

The *anaerobic lactic* system does not require oxygen to function (anaerobic). It does, however, produce lactic acid as a major by-product of energy production (lactic). The anaerobic lactic system is used in moderately intense activity lasting between ten seconds and two to three minutes. It is used when oxygen is in short supply or when there is a complete lack of oxygen.

The aerobic system

The aerobic energy system takes in, transports and uses oxygen. It requires the presence of oxygen to function. It is the main source of energy for events lasting longer than three to four minutes. The aerobic energy system is used for moderate intensity exercise and is developed and maintained through cardiovascular exercise, such as cycling, running, swimming, kayaking and rowing. Cardiovascular exercise stimulates the cardiovascular system (heart and blood vessels) and is, quite simply, any exercise that increases heart rate. It is also called cardio-respiratory exercise because it improves the ability of the heart and lungs to deliver oxygen to the working muscles.

The distance vs duration debate

Many athletes and coaches preach duration rather than distance when quantifying training. The reasoning behind this is that by training for duration rather than distance, you can avoid having to push yourself over a specific distance when you are tired. You simply train more slowly when tired, and still complete your workout. This may help prevent injury and overtraining.

There is, however, an argument for the use of distance. After all, if you are going to race over a specific distance, you have to cover it no matter how long it takes – no excuses! For this reason, particularly when training for longer races, it is sometimes better to use distance for your training.

I believe that both duration and distance should be used, for this provides more information (but don't become one of those 'crazies' who have to beat their previous time over the distance every time!). For example, when you do a workout over a set distance, don't look at your stopwatch. At all! Afterwards, however, total time or lap times can be compared against distance. You can then evaluate your workout and condition by considering the following:

- if you complete the distance in the usual time at the usual heart rate, things are good;
- if you complete the distance in a faster time at the same or a lower heart rate, things are even better – you are getting fitter;
- if you complete the distance in a faster time but at a higher heart rate, you are exercising too hard;
- if you complete the distance in a slower time at the same heart rate or a higher heart rate, you are too tired.

By combining distance and duration you can gain a lot more information on training than you can by just exercising to a set distance or duration. The question should not be whether to use distance or duration to quantify your training, but what is the most effective way to train. The answer then becomes simple: a combination of distance and duration is best.

Planning for adventures and simulating race conditions

During base work and the off-season particularly, plan exciting training sessions. Be adventurous rather than sticking to the same old training routes. And take friends with you so training also becomes a social occasion. This can help keep you fresh and enthusiastic.

During the speed phase you should start simulating race conditions, intensities and environments. If you can train on the course you will race on, do so. But don't train on the course every day as boredom can set in! Training on the course will help you to handle the course conditions better, improve pace judgement and make you aware of any special considerations that the course may require in racing.

Training should be simple to understand and enjoyable to do. If it is both these things, then you are well on the way to success. Indeed, training should be looked on as a personal adventure that is fun, challenging and rewarding. Perhaps above all else, training should let you look through 'the window of your potential' and see that the only limits you have are those you place on yourself.

Goal setting

Before you start planning your programme in more detail, you need to work out exactly what you want to achieve. Goal setting is one of the most effective training principles around. In a book by Mark McCormack titled *What They Don't Teach You In Harvard Business School*, he quoted a study conducted between 1979 and 1989 on graduates of Harvard's MBA programme. In 1979, the graduates were asked a simple question: 'Have you set clear written goals for the future and made plans to accomplish them?' Only 3 per cent of the graduates had written goals and plans, 13 per cent had goals but had not written them down and 84 per cent had no specific goals at all. A decade later, the researchers interviewed the members of that class again. They found that:

• the 13 per cent who had goals but not in writing were earning on average twice as much as the 84 per cent who had no goals at all;

• the 3 per cent with clear written goals were earning on average ten times as much as the other 97 per cent altogether.

The only discernable difference was the fact that the 3 per cent had goals, had put them into writing and had made plans to accomplish their goals. The same principle works in the world of sport – high performance requires three steps:

1 Setting your goals.
2 Working out how to achieve your goals.
3 Planning.

1 Setting your goals

The first step is to set your goals. These are important as they give you targets to aim for. Having goals also means you can start to move towards them: if you have a goal to work to, you are moving in a positive, predetermined, controlled direction. Goals power you up and set you off towards high performance.

2 Working out how to achieve your goals

Having a goal only means that you have a target to aim for. The next step is working out how to achieve that goal. Most athletes struggle with this step or miss it out; they can tell you what their goal is, but when you ask them how they are going to get there, you are met with silence. However, this step is crucial if you are to succeed.

Your plan needs to be more concrete than simply saying 'I'll do more mileage than before' or 'I'll train harder'. Instead, you need to look at what you are doing in both training and racing and highlight areas where you could improve. Start by identifying your mistakes and areas of weakness that cost you time or if you are embarking on a new sport for the first time work out what you need to know and who can give you good advice. Sit down with a piece of paper and start writing these out. You may find this difficult at first, but keep going. Give yourself at least an hour to compile your list. Don't see it as wasted time; this will be the most productive hour of training you spend all season as it will define exactly what you need to do. The clearer your goals and objectives are, the clearer the outcomes will be. It is impossible for me to overstate this point: setting up the method for achieving the goal is the fundamental basis for smart training.

Let's take the following list as an example for a triathlete:

1 I didn't get on the right person's feet in the swim.
2 I misjudged the tidal effects.
3 I needed to improve how I took my wetsuit off in transition.
4 My back got a bit sore on the bike, so I need to look at my bike setup.
5 I didn't climb the power climbs correctly.
6 I need to run better lines in the run.
7 I need to try to relax into the run at the start.
8 I also need to concentrate on running upright.

You then calculate how much time you could save by correcting these mistakes:

Objective	Time saved
Get on right person's feet in the swim	30 seconds
Judge tidal effects correctly	10 seconds
Improve taking wetsuit off in transition	4 seconds
Look at my bike setup	1–2 minutes
Climb power climbs correctly	10–15 seconds
Run better lines	20 seconds
Try to relax into the run at the start	15 seconds
Run upright	30 secs

Total time saved: 120–127 seconds (2 minutes to 2 minutes 7 seconds)

Setting out your plan in this way shows you clearly what you need to do: if your goal is to complete your next training session or race 2 minutes faster, you have a clear, easy, specific and concrete way of doing so. This is much more effective than simply saying, 'I want to go 2 minutes faster, so I'll train harder or do more training sessions', as the list will provide you with clear training objectives for each workout. This will allow you to get more out of your time and effort, and will save you countless hours of non-specific training. You might be able to increase the effectiveness of your workout by 150 per cent – imagine what you could achieve if you did this for every workout for a whole year.

3 Planning your training programme

A lot of people think a plan is a piece of paper that you have to follow, that there is no flexibility, that it's about complicated things like heart rates and all sorts of training details that cramp your style. However, I think a plan is a way of putting all your good ideas in one place so you can clearly see the steps required to get to your goal. It's no more complicated than that. It's not rocket science, it's just a method for turning a goal into a reality. It's a list of ideas about how to improve, set out in the right order and in the right quantities. Remember, goals are meaningless without some supporting process and plan underneath.

In summary, if you set goals, you generally move more rapidly and specifically in the direction of your goal. If you set up a supporting process by defining a list of objectives or steps that will lead to the accomplishment of the goal, you've defined all the things you need to do to achieve the goal. If you then put these objectives down on paper so that everything you need to do has a day it needs to be done on, is in the right order with the right quantities, and you can clearly see how you will achieve the goal, you have a training programme. Set this up and it will really make a difference. In three simple steps you will transform a goal into a reality (or at least more of a reality) and you will be one of the 3 per cent.

Understand what you are training for

Before you start planning your training, you need to fully understand the event in which you are going to compete. What you *think* you are training for and what you are *actually* training for may well differ, which can create big problems. If your perception of the event is inaccurate, your training for the event will be inaccurate and therefore your performance will be far lower for your effort.

Before you embark on your training journey towards your event, make sure you understand fully the nature of the event. Find a coach, talk to experienced people who have been there before, read about the event, watch documentaries on it:, do whatever you can to understand how the event works. Before you can even begin to think about your training you need to ask yourself what the event is really about. This doesn't mean the obvious, for example 'a triathlon is a swim, a bike and a run' – that's not what a triathlon is about.

For example, the limiting factor in most long-distance events is often your muscles, not your cardiovascular system. In a marathon it's your legs that tire first, not your lungs. You are not gasping for breath at the end of an Ironman, but your legs are very fatigued.

Endurance or strength endurance?

The most important thing to work out is whether you will be competing in an endurance or a strength endurance event. This will change the way you train for the event and will affect your success on the day: if it is an endurance event, most of your training will be long and easy, but if it is a strength endurance event, most of your training will be long and strong.

Below are some key points for specific events.

Ironman

- Ironman is a warm-up swim, a warm-up bike and a running race.
- 50 per cent of your effort goes into the swim and bike, and 50 per cent of your effort goes into the run on the day.
- Constant pace wins the race.
- Correct hydration and nutrition strategies are vital.

Marathon

- A marathon is a warm-up 30 km run and a 12 km running race.
- The first 30 km are about your physiology, while the last 12 km are about your willpower.
- Start at the effort you can finish with; even/negative splitting is vital (*see* page 00).

Adventure racing

- Knowing where you are is everything.
- It's not about you, it's about the team: how the team performs is how you will perform.
- Look after your feet at all costs.
- Look after your leg energy, with less effort on the uphills.

160 km bike race

- The first 15 minutes decides your time (because of the bunch you get into).
- Ability to place yourself in the bunch is crucial to preservation of energy.
- Set yourself up in the bunch for the corners and the climbs.
- Patience is key.
- Regular training bunch rides for cadence, hydration/nutrition and bunch etiquette are very important.

Here is an example. A cyclist could do a 160 km bike race and miss the bunch that they should have got into in the first 15 minutes because they were nervous to start faster at the start. They placed themselves nearer the back of the bunch rather than the top third and experienced the 'rubber band' effect for 60 km (37 miles) before they couldn't stay with the bunch. They were also too far back in the bunch for the corners and hills and also experienced the 'rubber band' effect slowly eliminating the strength from their legs.

When the next bunch caught up with them they were too impatient and went to the front and worked too hard and finally 'blew up'. They also didn't understand that riding in a bunch is a series of surges rather than a continuous effort and they hadn't trained for this and started to cramp in their legs. They nearly crashed bringing the bunch down because they were inexperienced at getting their water bottle out of its holder to rehydrate with so many cyclists around, decided to forgo drinking because of this and dehydrated reasonably seriously.

So the race result was very poor. This is despite the fact that the cyclist trained very hard for the event. If you don't know exactly what you're dealing with it's hard to get it right!

Understanding first, training second!

The key points mentioned above are the most crucial aspects to get right. How far you ride, run, swim or kayak and how hard you train are still important, but secondary to the key points. Keep them at the front of your thinking in training and the result will follow.

Once you have identified your goals and how to achieve them, you can start to look in more detail at various training principles to incorporate in your workout programme.

Training volumes vs intensities vs performance

Volume is the amount of training completed; intensity is the effort required for a particular form of training. Volume increases and decreases during training depending on where you are at in your build-up. Intensity, on the other hand, increases throughout your build-up, gradually in base but more rapidly during speedwork. Volumes of intensity increase and decrease.

Performance increases in a similar pattern to intensity, but remains low for a longer period of time and has a more gradual increase. During speedwork, performance begins to improve more rapidly and is at its peak rate of increase during the taper period (and to a lesser degree during compensation weeks at the end of mesocycles – more about this later). This means that despite all your hard training in base, you won't see the real benefits until very late in build-up. Figure 2.1 illustrates the changes in these three factors during a training programme.

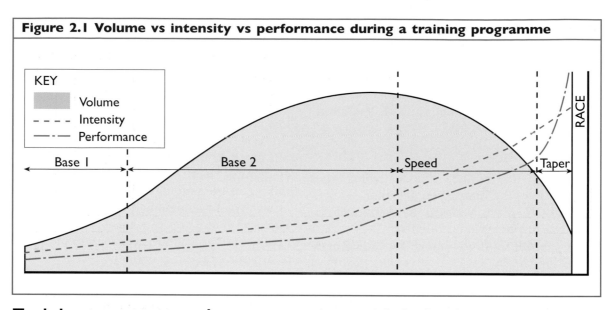

Figure 2.1 Volume vs intensity vs performance during a training programme

Training seasons and periodisation

Training is a form of stress. If it is done correctly, you adapt to that stress and become stronger. If it is done incorrectly, training wears you down and you can become 'weaker' – sick, injured, demotivated or overtrained. When you are any one of these things, you won't get the best out of yourself.

It is essential, therefore, that training is organised, in the true sense of the word. This means it balances work (stress) and recovery (active recovery or rest) – the two key ingredients of any good training programme. To help you achieve this balance, training is broken down into different phases. This process is called periodisation. Although top Olympic athletes sometimes work off a four-year training plan (e.g. Finland's Lasse Viren – double gold medallist at the 1972 and 1976 Olympics), for most athletes, the longest and most logical training period is a year.

A year can be broken down into three seasons. These are:

1 Off-season (transition)
2 Pre-season (preparatory)
3 In-season (competitive)

Figures 2.2 and 2.3 give examples of how a year can be broken down into three seasons based around race events.

Pre-season – preparatory phase (generally twelve to sixteen weeks)

As Figure 2.4 shows, pre-season training can also be broken down into different periods:

- Base training
- Base 1
- Base 2
- Speed training
- Taper and peaking

Very simply, base training builds a foundation of fitness, and speed training helps you adjust to the demands of racing. Taper and peaking allow you to perform at your best on race day.

Figure 2.2 The training seasons

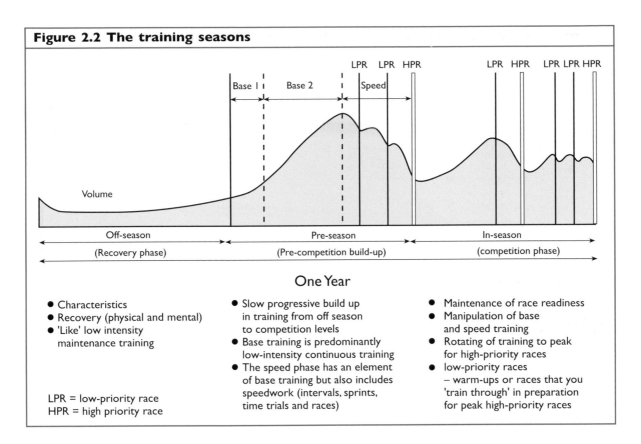

- Characteristics
- Recovery (physical and mental)
- 'Like' low intensity maintenance training

LPR = low-priority race
HPR = high priority race

- Slow progressive build up in training from off season to competition levels
- Base training is predominantly low-intensity continuous training
- The speed phase has an element of base training but also includes speedwork (intervals, sprints, time trials and races)

- Maintenance of race readiness
- Manipulation of base and speed training
- Rotating of training to peak for high-priority races
- low-priority races – warm-ups or races that you 'train through' in preparation for peak high-priority races

Figure 2.3 Seasons and periodisation for an endurance athlete aiming to peak once in a year for a major event

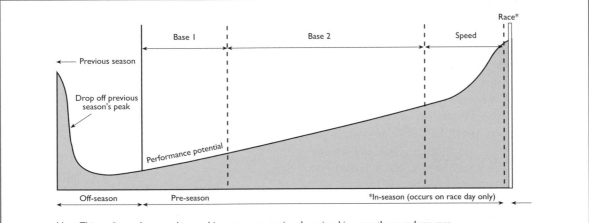

Note: This applies to Ironman, long multisport events, rowing championships, marathons, and any race that has top priority over all other races. It is also used when the race is so long that only one or two races (normally) can be performed per year.

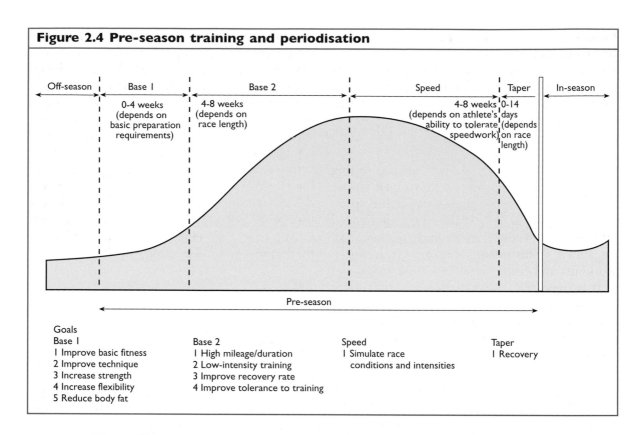

Figure 2.4 Pre-season training and periodisation

| Off-season | Base 1 | Base 2 | Speed | Taper | In-season |

Base 1: 0-4 weeks (depends on basic preparation requirements)

Base 2: 4-8 weeks (depends on race length)

Speed: 4-8 weeks (depends on athlete's ability to tolerate speedwork)

Taper: 0-14 days (depends on race length)

Pre-season

Goals

Base 1
1 Improve basic fitness
2 Improve technique
3 Increase strength
4 Increase flexibility
5 Reduce body fat

Base 2
1 High mileage/duration
2 Low-intensity training
3 Improve recovery rate
4 Improve tolerance to training

Speed
1 Simulate race conditions and intensities

Taper
1 Recovery

Base training (generally eight to twelve weeks)

Base training can last as long as six months, although it usually takes about two to three months. It really depends on how much time you have before the race or races you are aiming at, and how fit you are when you start base work. This phase of training consists mainly of high-mileage/long-duration workouts at a low intensity. These workouts are designed to improve your aerobic ability and muscular endurance.

As base training progresses you will find your tolerance to exercise improves – the so-called adaptation process. This enables you to recover from each training session more quickly. But, equally importantly, the base work will give you the endurance you need to cope with the increased intensity that comes later on in the programme.

Base training is divided into Base 1 and Base 2.

Base 1 – the preparation phase

The goal of this phase is quite simple: to get your body used to the type of exercise you are planning to compete in. For example, if you are a rower, you will become reacquainted with the boat and get back out on the water doing some easy technique work, if you haven't already been doing so during the off-season. Base 1 is also a good time to improve your strength and flexibility, refine technique and reduce body fat. The preparation phase is just that: a time that prepares you for the physical challenge that lies ahead.

Base 2 – the volume phase (mileage/duration)

During this phase, mileage is gradually increased. Training is still done mainly at a low intensity, although small amounts of speedwork can be done (particularly by experienced athletes). And *small* means *small* – you don't want to peak too early!

How much mileage should you do during this phase? That depends on how much you've done in the past. If you're new to the sport, then mileage will be less than for experienced athletes, and recovery from each workout will be slower. This means more time between workouts and fewer miles/km.

It is important to remember this when you are reading about a top athlete's training programme. It will have taken that athlete years of training to build up to that level. You copy them at your peril!

We all respond to training in different ways, and what works for one person may not work for another – that's what makes training such a personal adventure! Base training can be further broken down into sub-phases – easy, hills and sometimes up-tempo, which occurs more often at the start of speed. The first part of base is very easy training, followed by hill training during the middle to end of base. Finally, towards the end of base, up-tempo training is used to prepare your body for the speedwork in the speed phase (*see* chapter 4, 'Training Sub-phases'). Towards the end of Base 2, *some* up-tempo work (*slightly* faster than long slow distance) can be injected into the programme. This is to help the body begin to adjust to the real speedwork to follow. But remember this: base is *slow*! Training too fast during the base phase won't help you achieve race fitness more quickly and may even lead to injury, illness, peaking too early or overtraining. So be patient. Rome wasn't built in a day, and nor is fitness.

Base training is designed to allow you to cope with the intense speed phase to come. The better you are able to do the speed phase, the better your race performance is likely to be. Therefore, base on its own does not improve performance greatly (unless you race ultra distances), but it is essential to your later training. Some athletes put too much effort into their base training and arrive at the start of speed training tired. They then end up performing below full potential despite all the hard work put in. You could say they got excited a little too early! Be patient during base and remember the speed phase is the 'critical zone' – be ready for it.

The racing mentality

When training, leave home without it – your racing mentality, that is. It's often tempting when training with friends (and would-be opponents!) to start racing them. Don't!

During the base phase, it's vital you keep clocking up those miles/hours. You won't be able to do that if you train too fast, get tired and can't complete the next day's workout (a common mistake).

Some days, of course, long slow workouts are boring with a capital 'B'. On those days, and you will have them, it's okay to ease the boredom by doing two or three 'race-like' surges for a very short time. This applies mainly to training on the bike. To make sure these surges don't go on too long, decide where the surge will end before you begin it. If training with a group, make sure everyone regroups after the surge is finished; for example, sprint for a signpost and then regroup. These surges should be limited to one workout a week. And remember, there will be plenty of opportunities for competing with your training partners during the speedwork phase. Indeed, simulating race conditions during that phase can be a great motivator and plenty of fun. But in the meantime, don't worry about winning the local club run or ride.

Speed training (generally four to eight weeks)

After you have completed your base training it's time to add some speed to the programme. This will allow you to take advantage of the tremendous endurance you have built up in Base 1 and Base 2. The speed phase is the critical time. You need to be physiologically and psychologically prepared to put the 'hammer down' in the final four to eight weeks of training as this is where most of your performance gains will be made. Speedwork usually lasts about four to eight weeks, depending on your training history and how you cope with faster work. During this phase, training volume decreases and training intensity gradually increases. Towards the middle or end of the phase, some workouts will closely match racing intensity. As speedwork progresses, the body will adapt to the new stress being placed upon it. This will eventually translate to a faster race pace.

Certain aspects of your speed, for example acceleration/power, top speed, speed endurance and maximum steady-state pace, can also be worked on during this phase. This does not mean, however, that long slow workouts are neglected altogether. These still need to be done so that you retain your base conditioning.

Speedwork uses interval and sprint training, time trials and racing. It's very intensive (it often hurts like hell!) and therefore it must be managed carefully. Too little and you won't reach a peak; too much and overtraining can occur. The intensity of this phase also means there is more recovery time built into the programme. This time provides an excellent opportunity to refine technique. You must also contrast the intensities between speed training sessions and slow sessions. 'Creep' through your slow sessions as comfortably as possible so that you are able to 'hammer' the speed sessions.

Interestingly, some scientists suggest that for elite athletes a period of training overload ('superovercompensation', which would be overtraining if maintained for too long) should occur immediately before the taper, for example the third or second week before competition. This would only be done once or twice a year, however. Theoretically, a period of training overload enhances performance more than a traditional training programme in which overloading is not very severe. Why? Because the greater the training stress, the greater the body's adaptation to overcome it. This adaptation will, however, only occur if you follow the overload period with a long recovery period (the taper). Without this time to recover, overloading will become overtraining – the endurance athlete's 'death sentence'! (For more on superovercompensation *see* page 29.)

Taper and peaking (two to fourteen days)

A vital part of getting ready to race is freshening up. The tapering phase should happen before every race. The longer and/or more important the race, the longer the taper. Gradually easing back on the volume of training in the week or so before a race will bring you to a peak. The exact point at which you begin to reduce volume is determined largely by the event you're tapering for. For shorter events (around one hour's duration), two to four days is probably enough. For an Ironman triathlon, however, two weeks is probably best. A marathon taper is typically about ten days.

A common mistake in the tapering phase is to cut back on race-intensity work too soon. Only in the final few days should race intensity training be stopped altogether. By maintaining training *intensity* right up until the last few days before a race, you retain a better 'feel' for the effort that will be required on race day. The volume of training, however, is reduced.

Tapering is a very personal part of training and what works for you may not work for someone else. It's up to you to experiment and find out what suits you best. Some athletes, for instance, feel that they 'lose their edge' if they ease back too much, although it's much more common for people to race tired because they don't ease back enough. Similarly, some athletes feel they need speedwork right up to the day of the race; others find speedwork 'flattens' them for quite a while and so they avoid it as race day approaches. Either way, tapering always involves reducing training volume. And if you are unsure just how much to taper, have a longer rather than a shorter taper.

Figure 2.4 (*see* page 16) shows the four preseason training phases described above.

In-season – competitive phase (generally eight to twelve weeks)

This is when the serious racing begins! The competition phase usually lasts about eight to twelve weeks, with performance sustained at 90 per cent plus with one or two 100 per cent or 'full peak' efforts (lasting one day to one week) during this time. Alternatively, a competition phase may involve several peaks requiring a cycle of peaking and recovering over a period of about four months. A good training programme will let you excel at either a single/double-peak season or a multiple-peak season and examples are given in figure 2.5.

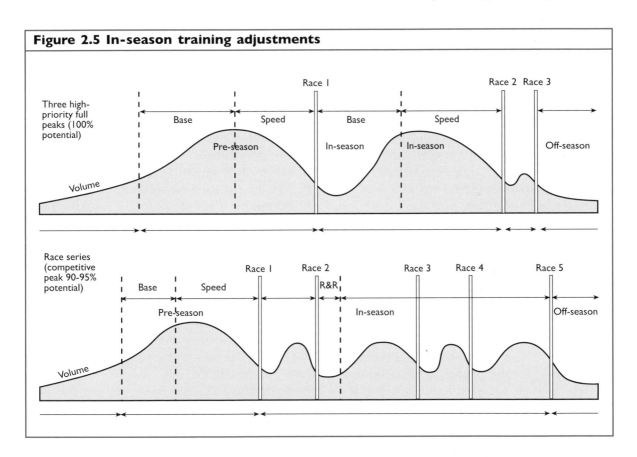

Figure 2.5 In-season training adjustments

Many athletes mistakenly believe they can hold a 'full' peak for three to six months. This is impossible. It can result in performance dropping away, injury, illness or loss of motivation, or all four. For these reasons, training during the competition phase must be closely monitored. This means carefully manipulating training volume and speedwork.

It's best to focus on only one to six high-priority races per season, with lower-priority races in between used as 'training'. Most athletes can only achieve a 'full' peak (100 per cent performance for a single race) two to four times in a season. These peaks often coincide with provincial and national championships and training is organised accordingly. For elite athletes, the peaks may coincide with national trials and world championships. In cases where the peaks are well spread out, such as a national series (multiple races spread over ten weeks), it will be necessary to achieve 'competitive' peaks throughout the season. These 'competitive' peaks require you to hold a high level of performance (95 per cent) over a series of races or a season. In this case, it is essential that fewer intensive training phases are inserted between races.

Speed training cycles and multiple peaks

These are normally used if you are in a race series. During the competitive phase you can set up peaks, or at least semi-peaks, from month to month. When trying to achieve multiple peaks it is essential that both the quantity (mileage) and quality (speedwork) are closely monitored from day to day and week to week. Too much of either will upset the programme and lower performance, or lead to injury.

These training cycles last about three to eight weeks. If the races are five or more weeks apart, a short period of base work with a small element of speed may be done immediately after races to allow for better recovery. Full speedwork can then be resumed. After racing, speedwork should not restart until recovery from the race is complete. And when you start speedwork again, keep the volume low initially. In the second week after a race, there is a gradual increase in mileage and speedwork toward the next race.

Multiple peak speedwork can be maintained over a competitive season that lasts two to three months. If the competitive season is any longer than this, a base training phase or an off-season becomes necessary again. And remember: too much speedwork can kill your season stone dead!

Off-season – active recovery or transition phase (generally four to sixteen weeks)

This phase usually lasts one to four months (four to eight weeks for elite athletes) and gives you a valuable chance to recharge the batteries (the 'recovery' bit) while still maintaining a reasonable level of fitness (the 'active' bit). Training during this phase is recreational (when you want, for example three times a week) and should be low intensity, low mileage. It's also a good time to work on technique or flexibility.

Off-season training doesn't need to be sport-specific either. Cyclists, for instance, could go mountain biking, swimming or running. As long as you are active it doesn't really matter what you do, although it is better if the activity continues to work your muscles and cardiovascular system in the same way your sport would. Elite athletes still need to spend a fair portion of their time doing their sport.

Overall, the key to the off-season is to make sure you begin the new season's base phase fresh, enthusiastic and ready to go, but also ready to build on last season's work and achieve a higher level of performance in the next season (*see* fig. 2.6). It's a fine line between being rested and being 'wrecked', but one which will become easier to judge as you become more experienced. Don't worry about losing *some* fitness – it's all part of a planned, well-structured programme. Besides, you and your body have earned a break!

The key to performance lies largely in how you do your off-season. Too much training in the off-season results in tiredness and lack of enthusiasm for training. This will affect your following build-up. Too little training means loss of the hard-earned performance gains from last season. The result is less improvement in your following build-up. If you do a little training in your off-season you will maintain some of the gains in performance from your previous season resulting in greater improvements in the following year. Your off-season can help or hinder your performance improvement from year to year.

Training cycles

Day to day: microcycles

A microcycle is used to maximise training on a day-to-day, workout-to-workout basis by balancing your training. The greater the recovery between workouts the more effective they become and the more progress you make. This can be achieved by using a hard/easy/hard/easy approach to training. As you get fitter, the harder sessions can, of course, become harder. Hard in base means more distance/duration; hard in speed means more speedwork. Intensity remains the same.

It is important that the hard sessions within a microcycle are not all of the same type of workout; that is, your hard sessions should rotate through long workouts, hill work, speedwork, and so on. If, however, you are training in a number of disciplines (running, cycling, swimming, kayaking), make sure similar workouts in the same discipline are kept apart. For example, long swims should not be done two sessions in a row. The key is to balance your training stress throughout the week. For a duathlete, a long run might be done in the middle of the week, so a long bike should be done at the end of the week. Similarly, a run speed session might be completed on Monday, and a bike speed session on Thursday.

Microcycles generally last 7, 14 or 21 days. For obvious reasons, the seven-day cycle is the

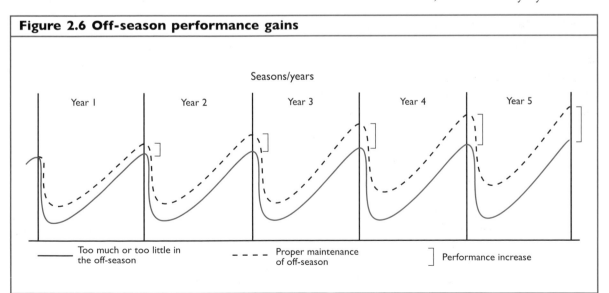

Figure 2.6 Off-season performance gains

Seasons/years

Year 1   Year 2   Year 3   Year 4   Year 5

——— Too much or too little in the off-season
- - - - Proper maintenance of off-season
] Performance increase

most common (*see* tables 2.2(a) to 2.7(b) for examples).

The microcycle can be changed during the racing season with hard sessions mid-week and easy sessions towards the end of the week as part of the taper for Saturday/Sunday racing. You may require more rest before or after an intense workout (such as speedwork), and this then dictates whether the preceding and following workouts are in the morning or afternoon.

The schedule in table 2.1, as an example, allows for longer rests after speed sessions.

Table 2.1	Microcycle morning and afternoon adjustments					
Mon	Tues	Wed	Thurs	Fri	Sat	Sun
a.m.	a.m.	p.m.	a.m.	D/O	a.m.	p.m.
Easy	Speed	Hills	Easy		Speed	Long

Table 2.2(a)	Microcycle for cycling and mountain biking – base phase					
Mon	Tues	Wed	Thurs	Fri	Sat	Sun
Easy	Hills	Easy	Hills	D/O	Long	Long
E	H	E	H	E	H	H

Table 2.2(b)	Microcycle for cycling and mountain biking – speed phase					
Mon	Tues	Wed	Thurs	Fri	Sat	Sun
Easy (Hills)	Ints	Ints	Easy	D/O	Race	Long
E	H	H	E	E	H	H

Table 2.3	Microcycle for triathlon – base and speed phases					
Mon	Tues	Wed	Thurs	Fri	Sat	Sun
Swim		Swim		D/O	Swim	
	Bike (Hills		Bike (S)	D/O		Bike (Long)
Run (S)		Run (Long)		D/O	Run (Hills)	

Table 2.4 — Microcycle for multisport – base and speed phases

Mon	Tues	Wed	Thurs	Fri	Sat	Sun
Run (Long)		Run (S)		D/O	Run (Hills)	
	Bike (Hills)		Bike (Long)	D/O	Bike (S)	
	Kayak (S)	Kayak (R)		D/O		Kayak (Long)

Table 2.5 — Microcycle for running (10km and marathon) – base and speed phases

Mon	Tues	Wed	Thurs	Fri	Sat	Sun
Easy	Med (Ints)	Easy	Med (Long)	D/O	Med (Ints)	Long
E	H	E	H	E	H	H

Table 2.6 — Microcycle for duathlon – base and speed phases

Mon	Tues	Wed	Thurs	Fri	Sat	Sun
				D/O	Run (Hills)	
	Bike (Hills)		Bike (S)	D/O	Bike (Long)	Bike (Long)
Run (S)		Run (Long)		D/O	Run (E)	Run (E)

Table 2.7(a) — Microcycle for rowing – base phase

Mon	Tues	Wed	Thurs	Fri	Sat	Sun
Tech	Med	Tech	Med	D/O	Long	Long
	Land		Land		Land	Land
E	H	E	H	E	H	H

Table 2.7(b) — Microcycle for rowing – speed phase

Mon	Tues	Wed	Thurs	Fri	Sat	Sun
Tech	Ints	Ints	Tech	D/O	Race	Long
E	H	H	E	E	H	H

Key to tables 2.2(a) to 2.7(b): E = easy; H = hard; Ints = intervals; Tech = technique; D/O = day off; Med = medium; Land = land-based training; S = speed; R = resistance

Week to week: mesocycles

A mesocycle is used to maximise training on a week-to-week basis and has a built-in recovery period to compensate for several weeks of long and/or intense training. This period usually lasts a week and is called a 'compensation week'. Mesocycles should occur regularly in the training programme, for example every second to fifth week, even during base training. These help you to steer clear of cumulative fatigue which, as the name suggests, can wear you down.

A mesocycle helps to keep you healthy and motivated: a great way to start the next period of hard training. It also allows for more improvement than a continuous build-up because of the adaptation to training that occurs when an easy period follows a hard period. Figure 2.7 gives examples of mesocycles to suit different types of athletes.

Most athletes have an easy week every third or fourth week, although some prefer alternating hard and easy weeks. Others, of course, can handle weeks and weeks of hard training without a break, but these athletes are few and far between and often perform at less than their potential because they never freshen up (*see* fig. 2.8).

Mesocycles are longer (five to six weeks) in early season base training due to the low training intensities, and shorter (three to four weeks) during the intense speedwork and competitive season.

Year to year: macrocycles

Macrocycles are used to plan the broad aspects of your training programme. This allows you to set out your training periods, training goals, and race priorities. As we have seen, this involves breaking down the year into three major seasons: off-season (active recovery), pre-season (base and speed training), and in-season (competition). These phases provide for seasonal/yearly recovery by including an easy period and a hard period in the training/competition cycle. Once you have established your macrocycles, you can slot in your mesocycles (week-to-week/month-to-month planning) and your microcycles (day-to-day planning).

Performance levels during competition build-up

Britain's great marathoner Ron Hill once said: 'A distance runner wakes up tired, and goes to bed tired.' Even with mesocycles this is, to some extent, both true and unavoidable for all endurance athletes.

In the build-up phase, 'cumulative fatigue' means you will always be training slightly tired – a natural side-effect of the body's adaptation to increasing training stress. This tiredness, however, needs to be carefully monitored.

This is the time when you must have faith in your training programme, because there seems to be a lot of hard work and little obvious reward. Once you start doing the lower mileages towards the end of the speed phase, you will feel less fatigue and your performance will tend to improve. Being slightly tired means you won't be breaking any world records in training. That's okay – they can wait until you start racing!

Alternative training cycle recovery strategies

In multisport and triathlon training, one effective strategy is to emphasise one discipline per week. The other disciplines are still done, but at a lower training volume. For example, in a three-sport discipline such as triathlon, swimming, cycling and running are emphasised on different weeks. This allows recovery from the mileage and intensity of each of the disciplines. Rotating the emphasis in this way may also be

2.7 Examples of mesocycles for the speed phase of training prior to competition

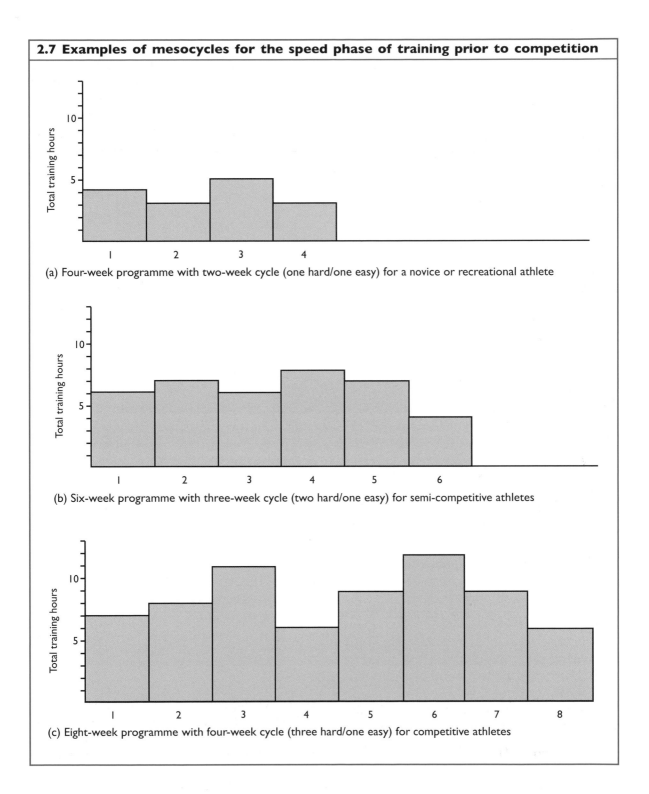

(a) Four-week programme with two-week cycle (one hard/one easy) for a novice or recreational athlete

(b) Six-week programme with three-week cycle (two hard/one easy) for semi-competitive athletes

(c) Eight-week programme with four-week cycle (three hard/one easy) for competitive athletes

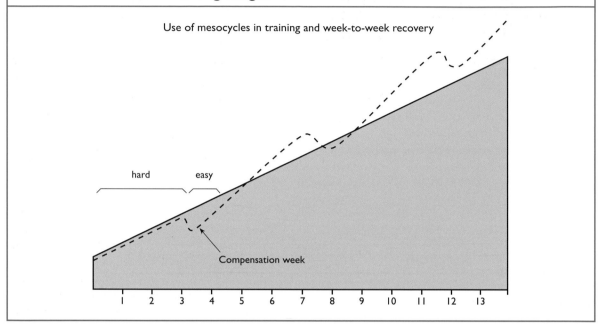

Figure 2.8 Use of mesocycles in training and week-to-week recovery. The dotted line indicates the variation in training volume (3 hard build-up weeks, 1 compensation week). The straight line indicates the continuous build-up method, which results in more chance of overtraining and generally results in less training being completed because of cumulative training fatigue

Use of mesocycles in training and week-to-week recovery

hard   easy

Compensation week

1 2 3 4 5 6 7 8 9 10 11 12 13

more convenient in terms of regular work, education or family commitments. For example, if your work takes you out of town and away from a pool for a few days every third week, this type of programme can easily accommodate this.

The schedule in table 2.8 shows how a 12-week triathlon programme may look with the emphasis alternating between the three disciplines.

Alternating the training emphasis in this way is an effective recovery strategy, similar in effect to a mesocycle. A mesocycle is probably best as it allows a complete recovery week, but this 'alternating strategy' may be useful for some athletes.

Table 2.8	12-week triathlon training programme										
Week	1	2	3	4	5	6	7	8	9	10	11	12
Swim	H	E	M	E	H	E	M	E	H	E	M	E
Bike	M	H	E	E	M	H	E	E	M	H	E	E
Run	E	M	H	E	E	M	H	E	E	M	H	E

Key: H = hard; M = medium; E = easy.

RECOVERY, TRAINING INTENSITIES AND HEART RATES

3

More isn't better

When training for a major competition or a series of major races, it is important to understand the aims of training. Large amounts of very intense training or high mileage training on consecutive days can be detrimental to performance if the body doesn't recover between workouts. This, as has been mentioned, can lead to overtraining and injury. It is important, therefore, that the training is balanced with adequate rest and recovery.

Balanced training ensures the body recovers after each workout. Only then will the body be able to adapt to a gradually increasing workload. High training volumes are only worthwhile if you can cope. Of course, as you become fitter, recovery periods shorten. But these periods remain as critical as the workouts themselves. Why? Because training, alone, does not improve performance. Rather: Training PLUS adequate recovery improves performance! This principle should guide your training at all times.

Recovery – 'The forgotten edge'

Too many endurance athletes get 'hung up' on mileage. They think that the more you train, the stronger, faster, and fitter you get. It is not as simple as that. If it were, there would be no need for books on training principles. The winners would simply be those who trained the most. Fortunately, endurance training is a lot more interesting than that. This does not mean, of course, that you can get away with a couple of

hours of training a week if you want to be successful. If you want to run a marathon, complete an Ironman or finish a cycle tour, then you will have to complete a certain minimum volume of training to do so. When the 'more is better' mentality takes over, the aspect of training most neglected is *rest*. Without rest and recovery you will not improve. This is hard for many endurance athletes to accept (even after repeated bouts of injury, illness and poor performance).

One 'problem', of course, is that endurance athletes tend to have a very, very strong work ethic. They also seem to get an 'attack of the guilts' if they think they are taking it easy. These 'guilts' may reflect a lack of knowledge concerning training, and/or a lack of confidence in their programme.

The key to improvement is not how much training you can do, but *how much training you can recover from*. That is what you should be thinking about when planning your training. A one-hour session that you don't fully recover from before the next workout will mean part of that next workout has been wasted. This is because insufficient recovery means the body has not been able to fully adapt. So, remember, *rest* is training too. Get into it!

Recovery strategies to boost performance

Your training is limited by two factors: how much you can do, and how quickly you can recover. These factors are obviously related and are very important in physically intense and endurance sports. Here are some ways to help recovery.

Warm-downs

These are particularly important after intense workouts such as strength and speed training. Warm-downs elevate heart rate slightly, increasing the blood flow to muscles. This helps to flush by-products such as lactic acid out of the muscles, providing a faster recovery than if you just stop training or competing 'cold'. The length of the warm-down is determined by the intensity of the workout. The more intense the workout, the longer the warm-down (15 to 30 minutes is appropriate most of the time). Of course, for low-intensity workouts (easy runs/ easy bikes), the beginning and end stages of the session are used as a warm-up and warm-down respectively; that is, you start off easy and you ease down towards the end of the workout.

Warming down after a race will certainly help ease post-race soreness and aid recovery. Of course, the temptation after a race is to stop dead. A good way to overcome this is to warm down with friends or opponents. It's a great time to find out what happened up front or behind you, and share in the black humour that athletes seem to enjoy after racing hard. Just make sure the warm-down is very easy!

Fluid replacement

This is essential! Excess fluid loss during training will reduce the quality of the workout and slow recovery. Even mild dehydration will take 24 to 36 hours to reverse, and will impair the next day's workout. Clear urine indicates you have rehydrated. Note, though, that if you are on multivitamins, your urine may not be clear even when you are rehydrated. It is essential (that word again) that you consume water before, during and after training and racing, or better still, a sports drink containing glucose polymers to replace energy as well (*see* chapter 12).

Nutrition

If you're training hard, you need to eat a balanced diet. This means ensuring your energy output needs (training) are matched by your energy input requirements (diet).

Finding the right dietary mix of carbohydrate, protein and fat is vital. If you are unsure whether your diet is meeting your needs adequately, consult a sports dietician. Generally, your diet should be high in carbohydrate (complex sugars in foods like bread, pasta, potatoes) and low in fat. Eating high-carbohydrate food immediately after training (within one to two hours) aids recovery significantly. For more on nutrition *see* chapter 12.

Sleep

Different people need different amounts of sleep. But for the athlete in training, eight hours a night is probably a good target to aim for. Perhaps more importantly, a constant sleep pattern is essential for recovery.

Before competition, it is the previous three to five nights' sleep that count, not the night before – which is just as well as nerves can sometimes make it difficult to sleep soundly the night before a race. This problem can be compounded if you are sleeping away from home.

Alternative activities as active recovery

Doing things other than the sport you compete in can be a great way to stay active, recover from competition and maintain your enthusiasm. Golf and walking seem to be particular favourites. For a runner or cyclist, easy swimming might do the trick.

Massage

Massage is one of the most underrated ways to look after muscles and prevent injuries. It also helps improve performance by promoting faster recovery from workouts – cyclists in the Tour de France use their end-of-the-day massage to hasten recovery from each day's racing.

Massage increases blood flow to the muscles, promoting the faster removal of by-products. This improves flexibility by reducing the 'tightening up' experienced after training and racing.

Knots of scar tissue are also broken up by massage. These knots are sites of potential injury as they adhere to the muscle, preventing smooth contraction.

For most athletes, a massage every week or two is sufficient to keep the muscles in good working order. Make sure you find a masseur who suits your needs and who is experienced in dealing with sportspeople (your fellow athletes will be able to recommend someone).

Relaxation baths, spas, saunas

If used properly, both spas and saunas seem to speed recovery by promoting relaxation and passive blood flow to the muscles and removing by-products. Just don't stay in them too long (especially the day before a race) as they can lead to dehydration and tiredness. Alternatively, ice baths are found to be beneficial for some athletes.

If you are in a 'leg sport', such as running or cycling, just putting your legs in a spa may be as effective as completely soaking the body, and less likely to induce fatigue. Hot water bottles on specific areas of the body can also be beneficial.

Overcompensation

Overcompensation is the physiological reaction of your body to training. It is, in a sense, an overreaction by the body to the stress placed upon it through training. This overreaction (adaptation) enables the body to cope with greater and greater training loads. This leads to improvements in performance (*see* fig. 3.1). This theory, that work and rest determine performance, is the basis for the use of training cycles.

Superovercompensation

Superovercompensation, apart from being the longest word in this book, is the same as overcompensation, only more so. Superovercompensation involves subjecting the athlete to greater training loads or stresses than is usual. This

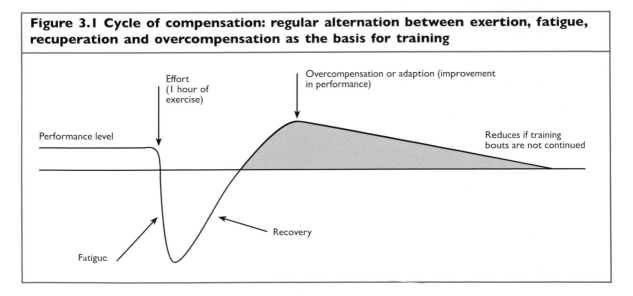

Figure 3.1 Cycle of compensation: regular alternation between exertion, fatigue, recuperation and overcompensation as the basis for training

results in a 'superoverreaction' or 'overadaptation' to the training load. Superovercompensation puts the athlete into a mildly overtrained state for a short time (a few days). As long as this period is only brief, adverse effects and overtraining can be avoided.

This technique seems to be most effective in sports where muscular stress is low, as in cycling and swimming. Runners need to be particularly careful when adopting superovercompensation as a training technique because the risks of injury are high. Instead of running more, runners may choose to add cycling to their programme in order to create the superovercompensation effect.

Inexperienced athletes should not attempt superovercompensation as it is a physiologically and psychologically severe form of training. Nor should superovercompensation be used more than once during a build-up. One bout of superovercompensation before tapering is most effective. Superovercompensation is most effective one to three weeks before a peak race. If done correctly it will produce a maximum peak above that of a traditional build-up (*see* fig. 3.2).

Small bouts of overcompensation may work every third, fourth or fifth week immediately before an easy week. In terms of daily training this could look something like the four-week schedule shown in table 3.1, which is also illustrated in figure 3.2.

Maintenance

If you do a one-hour workout and then let your body recover, you get fitter. If your next workout lasts one and a half hours, after recovery your fitness level would improve again, and so on (*see* fig. 3.1, page 29).

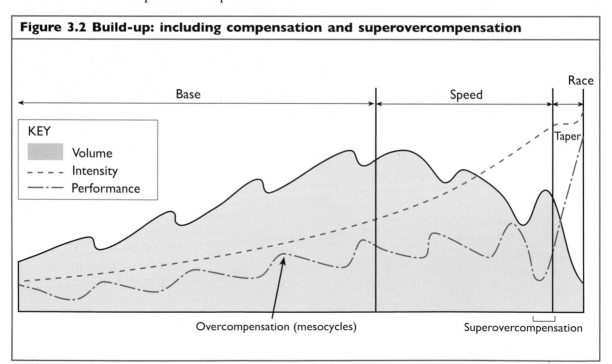

Figure 3.2 Build-up: including compensation and superovercompensation

KEY

▨ Volume
- - - Intensity
—·—· Performance

Base   Speed   Race   Taper

Overcompensation (mesocycles)   Superovercompensation

Table 3.1	Four-week schedule including small bouts of overcompensation						
Weeks 1–3							
Mon	Tues	Wed	Thurs	Fri	Sat	Sun
E	H	E	H	E	H	H
Weeks 4							
Mon	Tues	Wed	Thurs	Fri	Sat	Sun
E	H	H	H	E	H	H
Then back to week 1 again							

Key: E = easy; H = hard.

The law of diminishing returns

Here's an alternative situation: you do an hour of training and let your body recover, which makes you fitter. The next time you go out to train, you do exactly the same workout (same duration, same intensity, same type of training, same terrain, same conditions) – how much fitter would you get?

This is where the law of diminishing returns comes into play. The first time your body experiences a new workout, it will adapt significantly and rapidly. This is because the training stimulus is new and therefore a shock to your body; as a survival mechanism, your body will adapt in order to be able to deal with the same stimulus again. However, the second time your body experiences the same training, its reaction will be less as the stimulus is no longer new. The third time your body experiences the same workout, the reaction will be even smaller, and by the fourth time your body will have almost fully adapted to the workout. As a result, your body no longer reacts and your performance begins to plateau. After a while your body will begin to fatigue from the cumulative effect of doing the same thing over and over again and

your performance will start to deteriorate. In short, if you do exactly the same training over and over, there will be an initial training effect, then a maintaining effect, and finally an overtraining effect (*see* fig. 3.1).

Let's look at what this would actually mean in a specific training programme: a cyclist performing exactly the same 450 km of training week after week. At first he would see some performance improvements, but due to the law of diminishing returns he would see less and less improvement as time went on until the point at which he wouldn't get any fitter at all for each 450 km of training (*see* fig. 3.3).

After 8 weeks of riding 450 km each week, the cyclist has covered 3600 km in training. If the body adapted in the first three weeks and then plateaued, the cyclist wasted five weeks of 450 km of training, or a total of 2250 km. Therefore, at least 62.5 per cent of the cyclist's training was a waste of time. He could have progressed to 450 km/week later in his programme and timed his peak better.

A lot of endurance athletes constantly show their body exactly the same workout: they do the same ride around the same training circuit, they run with the same group over exactly the same course at exactly the same intensity, every week, week after week. As a result of not having to do anything new, their bodies don't adapt: no change in the volume, intensity or type of training means no performance gain. This is not training; it is *maintaining*.

Training vs maintaining

It's important to be clear about the difference between training and maintaining. As shown in fig. 3.4. Athlete B did not do as much training early on in the programme, and cumulatively did a lot less volume training than athlete A. However, athlete B still achieved his training goal of 16 hours for their peak training volume week, but because he hadn't done as many enormous training weeks in a row he was a lot fresher when it counted in the key weeks. In short, athlete B did less training, but timed his training correctly in order to peak at the right

time and ultimately finished the race faster than athlete A. Peaking is therefore about progressing at the correct rate: correct training plus correct timing.

Progression

If you don't change the type, volume or intensity of your training, you won't see any improvement. Even if you do large amounts of training, if you don't keep adjusting it to create a new stimulus, you won't improve. No progression, no progress, no performance!

Progression

Progression means adapting your training at the correct rate and in the correct order (*see* fig. 3.5). When you start training in a new build-up phase, your first objective is to get your *technique* working well. This allows you to become

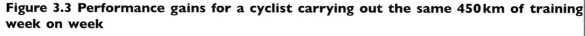

Figure 3.3 Performance gains for a cyclist carrying out the same 450 km of training week on week

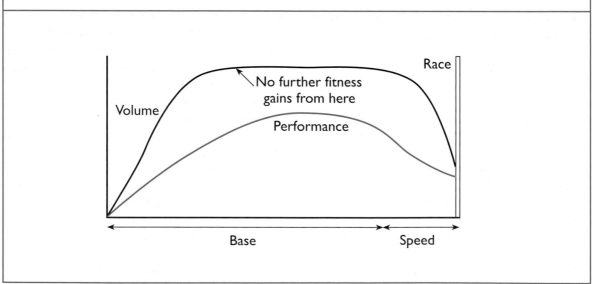

Figure 3.4 Training vs maintaining

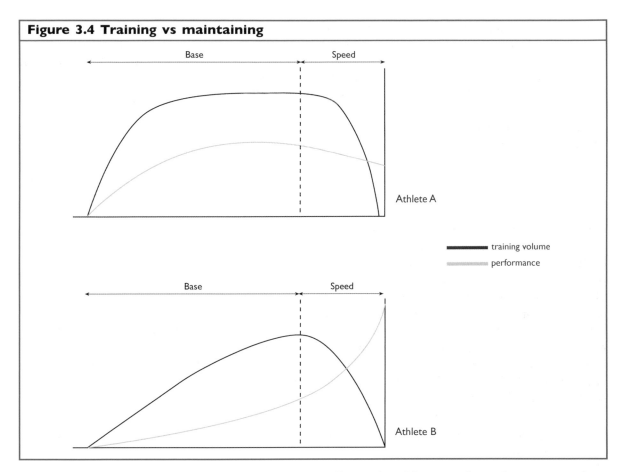

competent at the fundamental level of training. You must be able to perform the actions required by the event optimally: for example, for a triathlon you need to be able to swim, bike and run technically well.

Once you can do this, the next thing you need is *endurance*. This means being able to perform the action correctly for a long time (at least the duration of the event). Once again, taking triathlon (and more specifically Ironman) as an example, you need to be able to swim 3.8 km, bike 180 km and run 42 km, performing each action technically well.

The next aspect to focus on is *strength endurance*, which can be achieved by including a lot of resistance work in your training. You

will now be able to perform the action technically well for a long time with 'grunt'. Grunt is strength: the resistance you can move. In swimming, it refers to distance per stroke. Increased grunt means you can move yourself over a greater distance of water per arm turnover cycle, so you travel further for the same amount of effort. In biking, grunt is the gear that you can push; in running, it's your stride length.

Next comes speed, which is your ability to perform the action technically well, for a long time, with grunt, fast. Speed refers to stroke rate in swimming, pedal cadence in cycling and stride rate when running.

Finally, you need to get used to the conditions. This is about knowing the course well, having a good strategy and being able to handle the conditions appropriately.

Staying with Ironman as an example, by following this progression you would know the course well, have a strategy in place and be able to cope with the conditions; be able to swim 3.8km with a huge distance per stroke and an optimal stroke rate; then have a fabulous transition and bike 180km in a huge gear at a high cadence; then another great transition and run 42km with a long stride length at a high stride rate. These are the nuts and bolts of training and competition, what more do you need? The key point here is that if you're not focusing on the correct aspect or combination of aspects at the right time, then you're not training for the event. The training sub-phases

later in the chapter will show you how to correctly handle this.

Training intensities and heart rates

When someone asks you, 'How much are you training?', they usually want to know how far or how often you train each week. Seldom does anyone ask, 'How hard are you training?' Yet understanding the 'hardness' or intensity of your training is the key to understanding how a progressive, balanced training programme is put together. While novice and elite athletes may be poles apart when it comes to how fast they train and race, the intensity (not speed) of the work each group does in each phase of their training is the same.

Figure 3.5 Progression of training

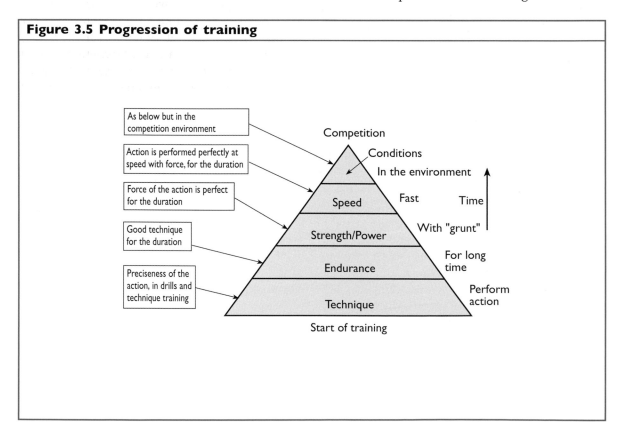

Training intensities have traditionally been categorised in many different ways. But they can easily be broken down into three basic types. Starting with the lowest intensity and moving up to the highest, these intensities are:

1 Low intensity (which can include active recovery, long slow distance, and up-tempo training).
2 Submaximal intensity (anaerobic threshold training).
3 High intensity (extensive and intensive sprints, and power training).

Low-intensity (LO) training is aerobic exercise (with oxygen) which can be performed for long periods of time. High-intensity (HI) training is anaerobic (without oxygen). High-intensity exercise (basically sprinting) can only be performed for brief periods before complete temporary fatigue occurs and you have to rest. Submaximal intensity (SM) training occurs at what some regard as the threshold or crossover between LO and HI training (*see* fig. 3.6).

Race pace (RP) training is a further intensity and fits into one of the three training types (LO, SM, HI), depending on the length of the race you are training for. This means RP will be slower (and less intense) if you are training for long races, such as a marathon, and faster (and more intense) if you are training for shorter races, for example a 10km road run.

Before discussing training intensities in detail, we need to look at how training intensity and heart rate together form a powerful training tool.

Heart rate – the athlete's 'revs'

Heart rate gives you a constant indication of how hard you are working: the higher the rate, the harder the heart is working to supply enough oxygen to the working muscles. Indeed, your heart rate acts like a rev counter on a car, telling you at what rate your 'engine' is ticking over. From this you can decide whether to work harder (increase the revs) or ease off (decrease the revs). And just as rev counters have a 'red

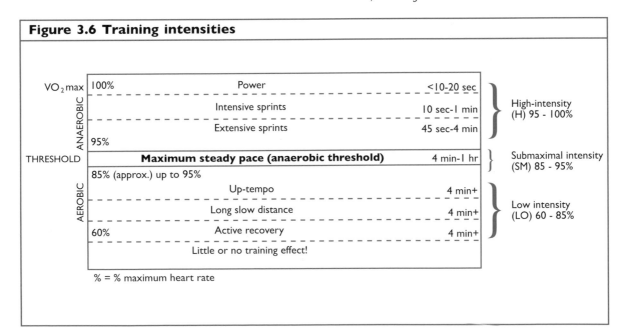

Figure 3.6 Training intensities

VO₂max 100%	Power	<10-20 sec	High-intensity (H) 95 - 100%
	Intensive sprints	10 sec-1 min	
	Extensive sprints	45 sec-4 min	
95%			
THRESHOLD	**Maximum steady pace (anaerobic threshold)**	4 min-1 hr	Submaximal intensity (SM) 85 - 95%
85% (approx.) up to 95%			
	Up-tempo	4 min+	Low intensity (LO) 60 - 85%
	Long slow distance	4 min+	
60%	Active recovery	4 min+	
	Little or no training effect!		

% = % maximum heart rate

line' marking an excessively high rev level, you too can work out a 'red zone' that will guide your training and racing intensity. Many heart rate monitors have a function that allows you to set it to 'beep' at different rates. This means you don't have to keep looking at the monitor to see if you are in the right 'zone'.

Knowing your training heart rates is a simple yet sophisticated method of controlling training intensity so that you maximise your training time and effort. But before you can do this you need to know what you 'idle' at – your resting heart rate.

Calculating your resting heart rate

Endurance athletes tend not to take things lying down, but in the case of your resting heart rate, you can make an exception. By measuring your heart rate* each morning for a couple of weeks, you will be able to establish your average resting heart rate. This is taken in bed, lying down, upon waking. If you wake up to an alarm, this can raise your heart rate slightly, so rest for two to three minutes before taking it. Make allowances if you have a busy day that day (anxiety), or if you need to urinate, as both may elevate heart rate slightly. Table 3.2 is an example of resting heart rates during a week. The figures are the numbers of beats per minute (bpm).

Calculating your maximum heart rate

Once you know your resting heart rate you will need to find out your maximum tested heart rate for each discipline you are training in: cycling, rowing, kayaking, running, swimming and so on. These heart rates need to be worked out when you are not tired from training, so a couple of easy days before each test is necessary.

To find your maximum heart rate, warm up for ten to fifteen minutes. Once warmed up, work out as hard you can for four to eight minutes with the last one to two minutes at maximum effort until you 'blow'! (Sprinting up a hill is useful, but do not make it too steep or leg muscle fatigue may occur before you reach your maximum heart rate.) Do this for each discipline, but make sure you are fully recovered between tests (allow a few days), otherwise the tests won't be valid and you won't be able to calculate your correct training intensities. Your maximum heart rate is the highest reliable heart rate reached during testing. This is best worked out using a heart rate monitor, but you can work out your heart rate manually as long as you do it immediately after the test. A maximum heart rate test can be dangerous, so if you are in any doubt about whether you can physically cope with it, see your doctor.

The simplest way to work out maximum heart rate is to subtract your age from 220.

Table 3.2	Resting heart rate over a week						
Day	Mon	Tues	Wed	Thurs	Fri	Sat	Sun
Heart rate (bpm)	56	54	55	56	54	56	57

Total heart rates = 388, divided by seven days = 55.4. This gives you an average resting heart rate for the week of 55 bpm.

*Using a heart rate monitor is the best way to get your heart rate. However, it is possible to take your heart rate manually by placing your fingers (not thumb) on your wrist (palm side) at the base of the thumb. Count the number of pulses for 15 seconds and then multiply by four. Alternatively, instead of using your wrist, you can place your fingers on your neck at the angle of your jaw.

Unfortunately, this not entirely accurate because of individual differences in heart size. Larger hearts beat fewer times per minute, so people with larger hearts will find it harder to reach their target heart rates using this calculation. This can result in overwork. Conversely, people with smaller hearts using the 220 minus age formula may find their target heart rates too easy to reach and therefore will not be working hard enough to meet their performance goals.

Karvonen heart rate calculation

By subtracting your resting heart rate from your maximum heart rate you can use the Karvonen formula to calculate your heart rates for various training intensities. These are usually expressed as a percentage.

For instance, submaximal (SM) intensity is considered to be an 85 to 95 per cent effort (0.85 to 0.95 for multiplication purposes). Thus, if your maximum heart rate (HR^{max}) is 196 and your resting heart rate (HR^{rest}) is 55, then your submaximal intensity range is worked out like this:

Karvonen formula:

$(HR^{max} - HR^{rest})$ – % exercise intensity + HR^{rest}

HR^{max} 196 – HR^{rest} 55 = 141

141 – 0.85 (85%) = 120

120 + 55 (HR^{rest}) = 175

---

175 is therefore the low end of your submaximal range. Repeat the calculation using 95 per cent and you get 189. This gives you a submaximal heart rate intensity range of 175 to 189.

When you begin training at your submaximal intensity, you should start off at the lower end of the range, in this case 175 to 180. As training progresses and you get stronger, you will be able to train more often at the higher end of this range, e.g. 180 to 189.

Ideally, your HR^{max} and SM intensity pace (also known as anaerobic threshold or maximum steady-state pace) should be worked out in a fitness testing laboratory. Mathematical estimates can be used, but these are not as accurate. Once you have got your HR^{max} and SM paces, you are then able to work out your heart rate ranges for the different training intensities, which are described in detail later in this chapter (*see* fig. 3.7). In essence, these ranges tell you how hard or easy to train in each phase of training. There is more on this in the sport-specific section later in this chapter.

Heart rates and what they mean

Heart rates at rest

1 A normal resting heart rate means you are fully rested and not fatigued.
2 An elevated heart rate, for example 10 per cent above normal, indicates fatigue and/or stress (e.g. 55+ for an athlete with a normal heart rate of 50). If it is only marginally elevated, continue to train and assess fatigue once training. Reduce training volume/intensity if required. If heart rate is only mildly elevated it is sometimes good to wait: you may be recovered and ready to train by the afternoon.

Unfortunately, resting heart rate is not foolproof when it comes to indicating your reaction to training stress. It can remain low even when you are tired (particularly in very overtrained athletes). Always subjectively monitor how you feel during training and when resting. If you feel tired, you probably are. Nevertheless, it is good to monitor heart rate during training. The orthostatic heart rate check (*see* fig. 3.8) may help.

Figure 3.7 Karvonen formula calculations

$HR^{max} - HR^{rest} - \%$ exercise intensity $+ HR^{rest}$
$HR^{max} =$ maximum heart rate
$HR^{rest} =$ resting pulse
% exercise intensity (see below)

Your maximum heart rate: .... (either by physical test or 220 – age)

Your resting heart rate: .... (in bed lying down on waking)

Fill in the spaces in the calculations below, using the Karvonen formula to work out your training ranges for each intensity. Accurate training heart rate ranges are impossible to obtain; these percentages are designed only to give you an approximate level as a guide for your training.

High intensity (HI) – anaerobic = 95–100%

(a) (........ – ....) × 95% + ... = ...

(b) (........ – ....) × 100% + ... = ...

Your HI training range is (a) – (b) = ... – ....

Submaximal intensity (SM) – maximum steady-state pace/anaerobic threshold = 85–95%

(a) (........ – ....) × 85% + ... = ...

(b) (........ – ....) × 95% + ... = ...

Your SM training range is (a) – (b) = ... – ....

Low intensity (LO) – aerobic = 60–85%

Up-tempo = 75–85%

(a) (........ – ....) × 75% + ... = ...

(b) (........ – ....) × 85% + ... = ...

Figure 3.7 Karvonen formula calculations cont.

Your up-tempo training range is (a) − (b) = ... − ....

Long slow distance = 60–75%

(a) (........ − ....) × 60% + ... = ...

(b) (........ − ....) × 75% + ... = ...

Your long slow distance training range is (a) − (b) = ... − ....

Active recovery = less than 60%

(a) (........ − ....) × 60% + ... = ...

Your active recovery training range is less than (a) = less than ....

Figure 3.8 Orthostatic heart rate test

The orthostatic heart rate test is a measure of overtiredness and is determined by calculating the difference between the standing heart rate and the resting heart rate: a 5 to 10 beat difference is usual, while 15 to 20 beats indicates overtiredness.

1 Calculate resting heart rate
Heart rate is taken in bed lying down upon waking. If you use an alarm, you must lie quietly for several minutes before taking your pulse. Try to take it lying in the same position every morning and note that a need to urinate may raise your heart rate slightly. Take this over a full minute.

HR^{rest} = ...

2 Calculate standing heart rate
Taken as soon as you stand up out of bed.

$HR^{standing}$ = ...

3 Calculate the difference in heart rate
$HR^{diff} = HR^{standing} − HR^{rest}$

HR^{diff} = ...

Note: differences between standing and resting heart rates may vary more than stated; if this is the case, use averages.

Heart rates during training

Using a combination of resting heart rate, training heart rates and training speed you will be better able to check on your reaction to training.

1 Resting heart rate normal, training heart rate normal, training speed normal. This indicates training and recovery are well balanced.
   Message: Everything's fine.
2 Resting heart rate normal, training heart rate elevated above predicted level, training speed above normal. This is particularly likely during base training and indicates you are training too hard.
   Message: Slow down!
3 Resting heart rate normal, predicted training heart rate cannot be reached, training speed can't be reached. This indicates fatigue in major muscle groups, such as 'dead legs' in cycling; your legs are so tired that they are not able to take you to the speed/intensity that you are capable of in training when 'fresh'.
   Message: Abandon programme for the day and have an easy day, e.g. 'spinning' in cycling, or go home and have a day off. This occurs more often when you are doing speedwork, like intervals or sprints.
4 Resting heart rate elevated, training heart rate elevated, training speed below normal. This indicates serious tiredness.
   Message: Have a day off, you may be ill!
5 Resting heart rate normal, training heart rate goes from normal to elevated considerably above normal while training or racing, training speed constant or begins to drop.
   Message: You may be dehydrated. Be very careful.
6 Resting heart rate normal, training heart rate above normal, training speed below normal.
   Message: You are overtired.
7 Resting heart rate normal, training heart rate normal, training speed below normal.
   Message: You are tired or you have 'dead legs'.

8 Resting heart rate above normal, training heart rate normal, training speed normal.
   Message: You may be experiencing mild mental stress/anxiety. Be very careful.
9 Resting heart rate normal, training heart rate begins to drop and cannot be held in a long workout, training speed drops.
   Message: You may have 'hit the wall', or 'bonked'.
10 Resting heart rate normal, training heart rate slow to drop after an effort (e.g. interval) or after a workout, training speed normal or marginally below normal.
   Message: You are probably fatigued or over-trained.

Heart rates during racing

Heart rate monitors can be very good for working out or adjusting your race strategy. (Racing heart rates tend to be 5 to 10 bpm higher than in training, because of race hype.)

1 Heart rate drops significantly during the race. This indicates you:
- started too fast;
- had an inadequate taper (legs too tired to hold pace for duration of race);
- did not do enough base distance work (specific to race);
- were overtrained;
- 'hit the wall', 'bonked', legs 'blew up' in longer races.
2 Heart rate increases slightly during the race. This indicates you:
- started too slow;
- had an ineffective warm-up;
- did not do enough speedwork (specific to race).
3 Heart rate increases significantly during race. This indicates you:
- are dehydrated (drink lots of water and check for other signs of dehydration).

4 Heart rate starts and remains too high for the duration of the race. This indicates you:
- are too tired;
- are overtrained;
- are ill.

5 Heart rate 'jumps', or fluctuates greatly (150 to 220bpm), in the space of a few beats:
- check transmitter, battery;
- wet your skin and the electrodes more;
- check signals aren't being affected by someone else's monitor or overhead power lines;
- accept it could be a heart abnormality.
- *Stop* exercising and see a doctor as soon as possible.

6 Heart rate remains constant at usual race pace level. This indicates you:
- had good race preparation and good race pace.

Things to know about heart rate monitors

Remember: your heart rate monitor is a tool not a dictator.

1 You can't train at a specific heart rate constantly; it is almost impossible. Terrain, fatigue and heat affect heart rate significantly. Use the heart rate range as a guide. (Don't crawl up a hill just because your heart rate monitor tells you to.)
2 Heart rates take time to move into your training range (up to 5 minutes), particularly if training is quite intense.
3 Heart rates can drop significantly from the start of training as you become fitter. Reassess regularly.
4 Heart rates will differ between different sports – heart rates for running are higher than for cycling, and cycling is higher than swimming.
5 Heart rates are generally higher during racing. 'Race hype' artificially elevates the heart rate by 5 to 10 beats.

Types of training intensities

As described earlier, training intensities are divided into three types: low, submaximal and high. First let's take a look at the least intense of these, low-intensity.

Low-intensity (LO) training – aerobic (approximately 60 to 85 per cent training range)

LO training gives you basic aerobic and muscular conditioning and it will improve your ability to metabolise (use) fat as an energy source. LO training can also be used to aid recovery. LO training can be broken down into three types. These too have an order of intensity:

1 Active recovery
2 Long slow distance
3 Up-tempo

Active recovery occurs at the easy end of the LO training range, while up-tempo occurs just below submaximal intensity (SM) training. LO training is performed at approximately 60 to 85 per cent of your HR^{max}. The Karvonen method of calculating your LO training heart rate range therefore goes like this:

For 60%: 196 (HR^{max}) – 55 (HR^{rest}) – 60% (0.6) + 55 (HR^{rest}) = 140

For 85%: 196 – 55 – 85% (0.85) + 55 = 175

This gives you an LO training heart rate range of 140 to 175.

Most athletes will work at the middle to low end of this range (active recovery, long slow distance) most of the time until up-tempo training begins in preparation for speedwork. If you do not have access to a heart rate monitor or you don't wish to use heart rates as a guide to training intensity, LO pace can be described as an easy to medium effort (if you can't comfortably hold a conversation at this pace, i.e. you're gasping, then you're going too fast!).

Active recovery (up to approximately 60 per cent training range)

Active recovery (AR) is at the lowest end of the training heart rate range. It is only used in training to assist recovery, for example by removing by-products from the muscles, or when you feel tired. Light activity is generally better for recovery than no activity at all. AR should be used on those days when you feel too tired to do your intended workout. But if after 10 to 15 minutes of training you still feel tired, go home and rest! Further training on that day will do more harm than good. If you feel you need a day off altogether – take it (and forget about training until tomorrow).

Long slow distance (LSD) (approximately 60 to 75 per cent training range)

Most of your mileage work will consist of LSD, especially during base training. This is not a very specific intensity, just an easy conversation pace. The pace will improve as you get fitter. Most athletes need to remember the 'slow' part of long slow distance.

Up-tempo (UT) training (approximately 75 to 85 per cent training range)

This is an intermediate intensity that bridges the gap between LO and higher intensity training. It is used late in the base training phase to help get you ready for speedwork.

Up-tempo training can be performed continuously or in intervals. The intervals will progress from long and easy to short and fast as your fitness improves. It needs to be stressed that up-tempo intervals are much longer than the type used in submaximal/high-intensity training. An up-tempo interval can be 15 to 30 minutes long (with long rests) at the start of up-tempo training. This is because the intensity is relatively low. Two to three up-tempo intervals may be done in one workout towards the end of base training, or at the start of speedwork, depending on your race distance (shorter races have up-tempo at the end of base; longer races at the start of speedwork). The days on which you do up-tempo intervals should correspond to the days on which you intend to do your speedwork, once the speedwork phase is begun.

As you adjust to the small increase in pace that up-tempo training involves (compared to LSD), intervals will become shorter and more intense, particularly as you approach the end of base work. Once speedwork begins, up-tempo intervals are replaced by higher intensity intervals. The length of the intervals will then gradually be increased again. In many cases, particularly for races that are shorter than two to three hours, up-tempo training becomes redundant once speedwork begins (*see* page 77 for more information on interval training for speedwork).

The effects of low-intensity training

Base training improves basic aerobic and muscular conditioning (including muscular endurance), speeds recovery and increases your tolerance to training. These training adaptations enable you to cope with the speedwork to come (and they improve your hill climbing ability if you have trained on the hills – good for cycling and running, not so relevant for kayaking!). Low-intensity training also improves your ability to metabolise fat as a source of energy. This means you are better able to race over long distances with less likelihood of 'bonking' on the bike or 'hitting the wall' on the run. And that's got to be good for an endurance athlete!

Submaximal intensity (SM) training – maximum steady state/anaerobic threshold (approximately 85 to 95 per cent training range)

SM training raises your maximum steady state pace (often referred to as 'anaerobic threshold' pace) and increases overall endurance or fitness. SM training includes intervals, time trials and, in most endurance sports, low-key races. SM training forms a vital part of any training programme because it plays such a big part in improving your race pace.

These days, anaerobic threshold is a term frowned upon by some sports scientists. This is because there is no absolute threshold but rather a 'grey area' where your body moves from functioning at a mainly aerobic level (where most of your energy needs are being met by oxygen) to mainly functioning at an anaerobic level (you can't take in enough oxygen to sustain your current level of exercise intensity). Therefore, the term 'submaximal intensity' is used to describe training that corresponds with that 'grey area'. SM training is usually about 85 to 95 per cent of HR^{max}, although these percentages vary a lot depending on your conditioning and the phase of training you are in. They can only be determined effectively through proper fitness testing (*see* page 111).

SM training should be performed at or slightly below the maximum steady state level; i.e. in the example calculated on page 37, this would be 175 to 189. If you have not been tested in an exercise laboratory, use the Karvonen formula and progressively increase intensity (and therefore heart rate) as you get fitter. That is, start at 85 per cent of HR^{max}, and using a five to ten beat range only, progress gradually to 95 per cent. In simple terms, SM training pace is medium to hard. You should find it difficult to converse at this pace.

The effects of submaximal intensity training

Various types of SM training will improve steady state racing speed and improve muscle endurance. Time trials and low-key races will help you prepare physiologically, mentally and technically for racing. The mental aspect is particularly important because you need to get used to coping with race intensity (and the nervous tension that often precedes it!).

As time trials are hard work, you should only do them over distances that are about 33 to 50 per cent of race distance (for sub-three hour races). For a 10 km race, for instance, 5 km time trials are sufficiently long for training purposes. For triathlons with a 40 km cycle, 20 km time trials are appropriate. Even then, they will be very tiring and may hinder training for the rest of the week (*see* page 77 for more information on time trials for speedwork).

Intervals are an alternative form of SM training. These can be differentiated from high-intensity intervals by the fact that they are over four minutes in duration. As you get fitter, the workload (number and length of efforts) will increase and the rests will get shorter until you are performing at a high steady state pace for a long time with little rest. At this point you are virtually doing a time trial.

For endurance sports, intervals should be longer than four minutes to ensure you are exercising at submaximal intensity – less than four minutes and there is a danger the exercise intensity will be too high (anaerobic). Submaximal training is particularly useful for cycling (time trial events and long breakaways), mountain biking, sprint and standard distance triathlon, running, duathlons, multisport and rowing racing. Submaximal intensity training is the cornerstone of your racing speed.

High-intensity (HI) training – anaerobic (approximately 95 to 100 per cent training range)

HI training bears some similarity to SM training, but it also improves your ability to cope with sprinting (acceleration, top speed and speed endurance), sprint recovery (oxygen debt), and high levels of exertion. High-intensity training can be broken down into sprinting (extensive and intensive) and power (acceleration). The Karvonen heart rate calculation for HI training goes like this:

196 (HR^{max}) – 55 (HR^{rest}) x 0.95 (95%) + 55 = 188

To exercise at 95 per cent plus of your HR^{max} means sprinting. It is the only time in training you should let all the brakes off and go for it. To some extent, it is hard to define and monitor exact heart rate levels at this intensity. If using a heart rate monitor, it is assumed that heart rates must be above 95 per cent HR^{max} to have the desired effect. But it is better to use the duration of the sprint to control intensity. Why? Because in very short sprints your heart rate will not reach a constant, meaningful level. HI training pace can be described as hard to very hard. You should not be able to talk. Actually, even thinking should be difficult!

What makes up high-intensity (HI) training?

1 Extensive (EX) sprints (90 to 95 per cent effort/45 sec to 4 min duration)
These are long sprints and are used to condition your body to extended sprinting (speed endurance). Extensive sprints are very good for cycle racing, any multisport races that involve some aspect of cycle racing in a bunch (peloton), mountain bike starts, distance running and rowing.

2 Intensive (IN) sprints (100 per cent effort/10 sec to 1 min duration)
These are short sprints and are used to improve your top speed and speed endurance. This is effective for cycle racing, mountain bike starts and, to some extent, rowing. Intensive sprints are not as effective for the other endurance sports dealt with in this book, although both intensive and extensive sprints may, when done at the right phase of your training programme, improve leg speed.

3 Power (PW) sprints (100 per cent effort/ less than 10 to 20 sec duration)
This is used to develop explosive ability (efforts generally lasting less than 10 seconds) and is useful for cycling (to improve the 'jump' or acceleration). Power can also be effective for rowing. It is of little benefit to the other sports dealt with in this book.

High-intensity training improves your recovery from oxygen debt and your ability to sustain pace in oxygen debt (lactate tolerance). It is good for fast starts and finishes, it is also very good in cycling for pushing up and over hills, breakaways, sprint primes, sprint finishes and starts, and for bridging gaps between bunches. Acceleration, top speed and speed endurance can be developed separately or in combination, generally progressing from EX to IN and finally to PW. Overspeed (an aspect of HI: lighter load and a muscle contraction slightly higher than race pace) can also be used for cycling. High-intensity training levels need to be manipulated precisely at the right time to improve racing ability. Too much speedwork overtrains; too little speedwork undertrains (*see* page 78 for more information on sprints for speedwork).

Race pace (RP) training
Race pace training simulates race conditions and intensities. It conditions the body physically

and mentally to tolerate race pace. Which training intensity it fits into depends on general race pace. RP training is determined by your racing distance. The longer the race, the lower your RP. It is also determined by your fitness and ability. For this reason, it is difficult to calculate RP accurately. Nevertheless, it can be defined simply as this: race pace is the pace you feel you can maintain for the entire race.

RP can best be gauged by using a heart rate monitor with memory to record racing heart rates. This gives a clear indication of this training intensity. But note, it must be checked within four to six weeks of a major race. Although RP training should be done at this established level, pushing too hard (intensity too high) in this type of training will not improve racing ability. The transition from submaximal training to race pace training is made during the speedwork period. A combination of SM training and RP training should be used only in the last few weeks before peaking. In preparing for longer races (over three hours), a slightly different approach is used as SM training is used relatively less than RP training. RP training is also initiated before SM training.

Sport-specific heart rate monitor use

Time trial

The best way to race any form of time trial distance event is to maintain an even pace or effort. This enables you to use your energy resource in the most 'economic' way possible. Changes of pace or effort are expensive and drain your 'energy bank account' quickly. The even pace, of course, should be the fastest pace you can sustain for the entire race or time trial. This pace, for example, may be for a race of one hour at your submaximal (SM) or anaerobic threshold pace.

As described previously, your submaximal pace will have a corresponding heart rate (85 to 95 per cent of HR^{max}). Once you know this heart rate you can use it to help keep your effort strong and steady for an entire race or time trial. This is particularly useful when racing over hills or in windy conditions, as both situations contribute to heart rate fluctuations. It is worth remembering also that different disciplines produce different heart rates at similar intensities.

To find your target racing heart rates (as opposed to your SM training heart rates) for each discipline, you should do a time trial at a pace you think you could sustain for the race distance. Time trials are 33 to 50 per cent of race distance for sub-three-hour races, and 50 to 75 per cent for races over three hours. For example, time trials should be 2 to 3 hours for a 4 hour plus race; 45 to 60 minutes for a 1.5 to 2 hour race; and 15 to 30 minutes for a 30 minute to 1 hour race. If possible, try to do the time trial over a course similar to the one you will be racing over.

These time trials should be done every two to four weeks during speedwork, and they are substituted for another speed session (they're not an extra one!). Because of the lack of race hype, your heart rate in these time trials may be 5 to 10 beats lower than actual race pace intensity. If this is the case, the only way to obtain racing heart rates will be by racing.

If you are racing a lot, use the races as time trials. These time trials will give you a starting heart rate, for example 160 to 165. If you found this too comfortable, then next time out increase it by 5 beats. Keep increasing the heart rate until you can't hold it for the entire time trial. When this happens, drop back to the previous heart rate and retest. This will probably be your current racing heart rate. This method is especially good for working out the heart rate for long races. For shorter races, low-key races can be used instead of time trials. Be careful, though, that other training factors, such as tiredness or speedwork, are not affecting time trial results (*see* page 77 for details on time trials and speed training).

Cycling – heart rate/cadence link

When on the bike it is useful to link heart rate to cadence (how fast you're pedalling). This allows you to optimise gear changes as well as pace. Optimal time trial cadences are around 85 to 95 revs per minute (rpm). *See* table 3.3.

Using a heart rate to monitor effort on the bike is particularly useful for inexperienced cyclists, though notable improvements in performance have also been achieved by experienced riders. Inexperienced cyclists often push too big a gear, causing severe leg fatigue. End result? They end up 'legless' late in the race. This is because the lower the cadence (big gears), the more muscular the effort is. The higher the cadence (small gears), the more cardiovascular the effort is.

The optimal cadence, of course, lies somewhere in the middle; for example 90 to 110 rpm for a road race, 85 to 95 rpm for a time trial. It is important for triathletes and duathletes to understand this because not only will monitoring heart rate on the bike help your bike time, but the less leg fatigue you can incur on the bike the better you will go in the run.

Heart rate can also be used to check whether you have warmed up properly, and on the bike it can measure bike/rider efficiency, aero position, biomechanical variables, bike set-up, and the like, although each test should be done in identical conditions and at race pace. Heart rate can also be productively used in combination with new cycle computers that measure not only speed but also work (watts).

Cycling – road race

Aside from being used to maintain your SM pace (and an even effort), heart rate monitoring can be used to find out where in the bunch (peloton) you travel most easily. Heart rate can also be used to help you decide when to chase (heart rate low beforehand) and when not to chase

Table 3.3	Example of the heart rate/cadence link	
Optimal race pace heart rate (tested) = 170 to 175		
Optimal cadence = 85 to 95		
Heart rate	**Cadence**	**Analysis**
172	87	Excellent. Hold effort.
180	89	Heart rate too high; you are going too hard. Change to easier gear.
140	92	Heart rate too low; too easy. Change to a harder gear.

Note: You will need to watch heart rate and cadence constantly as both change as the course changes and you become fatigued.

(heart rate high beforehand). A low heart rate while in the bunch indicates you are fresh and strong and ready to attack. If heart rate has been high for some time, it is best to relax in the bunch until you recover. Finally, don't become a slave to heart rate, especially towards the end of races. Sometimes you've just got to go for it.

Cycling – stage race

In addition to the guidelines outlined above for road races, heart rates can also be used to monitor energy levels from day to day. For instance, if rest and exercise heart rate is as predicted or below on a particular day, the stage suits your strengths, and your legs feel fine, this might be the day to attack. If, on the other hand, your heart rate is high, then it would probably pay to sit in the bunch and wait for another day. Resting heart rates can also be taken each morning to see how well you've recovered from the day before (see previous time trial and cycling sections).

Multisport

The important consideration here is that each discipline will have a different racing heart rate, with a significant difference between upper and lower body exercises (*see* time trial section on page 77).

Mountain biking

Mountain biking is like cycle time trials, so a constant heart rate and intensity is desirable once the start is over and your position is established (*see* time trial section on page 77). As it is difficult to look at your monitor when mountain biking, make sure you get one that can be set to beep at different levels.

Running

Maintaining a constant pace is crucial when running. A heart rate monitor provides constant feedback on effort, as opposed to 'splits' which are often too infrequent to help with pace judgement.

Rowing

The best way to use a heart rate monitor in rowing is to strap it to the stroke in successive races. You can only use one monitor in the boat at a time as they transmit on the same frequency. The stroke is the best person to wear it as he/she determines pace. Use the memory mode to collect a number of time trial/racing heart rates two to three weeks before the major race, then assess what the race pace heart rates are for each 500 metres and work out the crew's race pace.

Generally in rowing, pace is constant, although the first and last 500 metres are marginally faster. Once race pace is known, the coxswain can indicate to the stroke whether to work harder or 'back off' to achieve optimal pace. However, it shouldn't be forgotten that you are racing and sometimes race strategy will override heart rate considerations.

Each rower's heart rate can also be assessed before the start of speedwork so that appropriate training intensities can be worked out (each rower will probably have a different racing heart rate). Heart rates could also be used to check rowing efficiency, for example inboard versus outboard ratio on oar, racing stroke rate. The aim, of course, is to achieve the fastest boat speed at the lowest heart rate.

TRAINING SUBPHASES

4

The training phases

As discussed previously, training for endurance sports can essentially be broken down into two phases – the base and speed phases. But that doesn't just mean slow and fast! Indeed, there are a number of training factors that must be addressed under the headings of base and speed. But before we look at what these factors are, and how they form the 'subphases' of training, let's briefly revisit the base and speed phases.

Base   – endurance/technique (Base 1)
           – strength endurance (Base 2)
Speed – speed

The base phase

The base phase is primarily designed to build basic sport-specific 'fitness'. It does this by increasing your tolerance *to* training, and by promoting faster recovery *from* training.

Base 1

Base training initially focuses on technique and endurance. This first period of the base phase is called Base 1. Base 1 is designed to get you conditioned to training. It provides basic fitness and gives you time to address any weaknesses, physical and technical, you may have. Examples of Base 1 training are:

- Cycling – pedalling easily for a long ride
- Rowing – rowing with half/three-quarter pressure on the blades
- Running – easy long runs

Essentially, Base 1 allows you to complete the race distance (or, for longer races, get close to completing the race distance).

Base 2

After Base 1 comes Base 2 – strength endurance training. This period of base training gives you the ability to apply more 'grunt' (strength, power, force) as you complete the race distance. Examples of Base 2 training are:

- Cycling – riding in a bigger gear (low cadence; on hills and flat ground)
- Rowing – rowing with some form of drag (e.g. bungy, rope tow)
- Running – long strides uphill, uphill bounding and stride outs

Strength endurance training involves the application of more and more muscular effort to training, through to the point where speed begins to gradually increase in speedwork.

Overall, the main purpose of the base phase is to allow you to do effective speedwork or, more accurately, race-specific conditioning, later on.

The speed phase

The human body responds to training stress by *adapting specifically* to that training stress. In order to prepare for the stress of racing, therefore, speedwork needs to more and more closely resemble racing intensities and conditions. Consequently, speed training generally follows this order:

- Up-tempo training (occurs at the end of base or start of speed training depending on the race length)
- Anaerobic threshold/maximum steady-state training
- Long sprints (if required)
- Short sprints, power and overspeed (in that order if these types of training are required)

To summarise: during the base and speed phases, training moves from endurance/technique to strength endurance to speed to peak (*see* fig. 4.1).

Now, let's look at the 'subphases' of training.

The training subphases

The nine training subphases are shown in figure 4.2. Note that there is a progression from endurance/technique training, through to sport-specific strength endurance training, through to

speed training. In other words, your training moves from less race-specific training to more race-specific training as your goal race approaches.

We can then apply these subphase requirements to specific sports and training programmes. Figure 4.3 illustrates the subphases for individual sports and events and how they relate to the two main phases, base and speed, of an endurance training programme.

Each of the nine subphases will now be described based on the graph illustrated in figure 4.3. The descriptions include sport-specific guidelines and examples of training weeks. The workout themes used in the training weeks are: (H) = hills; (S) = speed; (L) = long; (ML) = medium long; (S/H) = speed or hills; E = easy.

Base phase

All heart rates in the base phase are at long slow distance rates (60 to 75 per cent HR^{max}), unless otherwise specified.

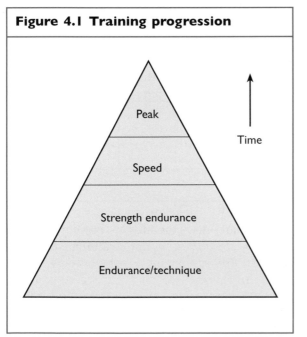

Figure 4.1 Training progression

Peak

Speed

Strength endurance

Endurance/technique

Time

Figure 4.2 Training subphases in relation to the main training phases of base (Base 1 and Base 2) and speed

Subphase		Period/Phase
1	Preparation (easy)	Endurance/ technique (Base 1)
2	Load	Strength endurance (Base 2)
3	High load	
4	Load/Speed	
5	Low speed	Speed
6	High speed	
7	Sprints (if required)	
8	Power (if required)	
9	Overspeed (if required)	

Figure 4.3 Explanation of subphases

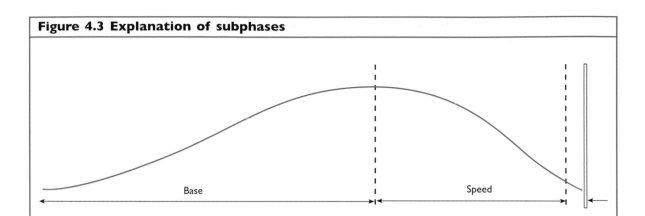

Subphase	1 EASY	2 LOAD	3 HIGH LOAD	4 LOAD/ SPEED	5 LOW SPEED	6 HIGH SPEED	7 SPRINTS	8 POWER	9 OVER- SPEED
Triathlon	easy	hills/pull buoy	hills, big gear hills, long stride, paddles/band	flat/big gear stride outs (bound) pull buoys	up-tempo	anaerobic threshold			
Duathlon	easy	hills	hills, big gear hills, long stride	flat, big gear stride outs (bound)	up-tempo	anaerobic threshold			
Multisport	easy	hills/ bungy	hills, big gear hills, long stride, bungy/rope tow	flat, big gear stride outs (bound) bungy	up-tempo	anaerobic threshold			
Running	easy	hills	hills, long stride	stride outs (bound)	up-tempo	anaerobic threshold	extensive sprints		
Mountain biking	easy	hills	hills, big gear	flat, big gear	up-tempo	anaerobic threshold	extensive sprints		
Rowing	easy	bungy	bungy/rope tow	bungy	up-tempo	anaerobic threshold	sprints	power	
Cycling	easy	hills	hills, big gear	flat, big gear	up-tempo	anaerobic threshold	sprints	power	over- speed

Period: Endurance/technique (Base 1).
Subphase 1: Preparation (Easy)

Preparation involves easy conditioning and occurs as you get back into a more structured training programme after your off-season. Preparation gets the body ready for what lies ahead. The preparation subphase is also a good time to look at problems (e.g. flexibility, strength imbalances, etc.) and continue work on rehabilitation if needed. Depending on your background and the amount of training done in the off-season you might be able to skip the preparation subphase. Alternatively, it could take many weeks if problems need to be resolved. In particular, technique should be emphasised at this time, especially for running, cycling, swimming, rowing, and kayaking. Preparation occurs at the start of Base 1 and can last zero to eight weeks (generally two to four).

Subphase 1: Preparation

Specifics: Light/easy conditioning in all sports
Effort: Easy conversation pace (50–60% effort)
Sports:
  Swim: Easy/technique
  Bike: Easy/small gears. Cadence 85–95 rpm if time trial or *Tri/Du/mountain biking*: 85–95 rpm for road cycling
  Run: Easy
  Kayak: Easy
  Row: Easy (½ pressure, low stroke rate: 18–22 strokes per minute)

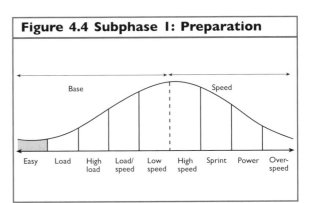

Figure 4.4 Subphase 1: Preparation

Table 4.1(a)	Training week in subphase 1 (triathlon/duathlon/multisport)					
Mon	Tues	Wed	Thurs	Fri	Sat	Sun
S/K (H)		S/K (S)		DAY OFF	S/K (L)	
	B (S)		B (H)			B (L)
R (H)		R (H)			R (H)	

Table 4.1(b)	Training week in subphase 1 (cycling/mountain biking/ running/rowing)					
Mon	Tues	Wed	Thurs	Fri	Sat	Sun
E	S/H	E	ML	DAY OFF	S/H	L

For **bold** workouts, use the form of training specified for each sport.

Speed phase

Once base training is completed, you are ready for the speed phase. Now the real work starts. You can begin to increase the tempo of your training. Everything up until now has been important, but the final weeks of the speed phase 'make or break' your chances of a top performance.

The following subphases are progressively combined into one to three speed sessions per week (1 = novice, 3 = elite) over the last four to eight weeks of the speed phase.

Sometimes racing over shorter distances is a better (more specific) form of speed training and can be substituted for a speed session. But remember: a race does not act as an extra speed session. Speedwork is very intense and demanding. Too much speedwork can quickly overfatigue you and destroy your build-up. Therefore, be careful. There is a fine line between too much and too little speedwork. As a rule of thumb, 10 per cent of your training in your biggest speedwork week can be at anaerobic threshold intensity or higher (or 20 per cent up-tempo or higher, and 80 per cent long slow distance).

Each of the following subphases is introduced progressively each week during the speed phase.

Period: Speed. Subphase 5: Low speed

Cycling, running

For cycling and running, up-tempo work marks the beginning of the conditioning work for speed. This form of training is faster than easy conversation pace but not as high as 10–60-minute-race pace. When cycling, for example, you should be riding fast (70 to 75 per cent effort) and feeling strong (i.e. Ironman/marathon race pace), but not 'hammering'. Because low speed training is only moderately intense, the interval periods can be quite long (10–20 minutes). This would occur one to two times per week and would be gradually phased in over a period of one to four weeks (generally two).

Subphase 5: Low speed

Specifics: Long intervals at up-tempo pace (Ironman race pace). You should feel fast and strong
Effort: Moderately difficult to converse (70–75% effort)
Sports:

> *Swim:* 600–1000 m intervals
> *Bike:* 10–20 min intervals
> *Run:* 10–15 min intervals
> *Kayak:* 10–20 min intervals
> *Row:* 10–20 min intervals

Training heart rate: Up-tempo rate (75–85% HRmax) for intervals; long slow distance rate (60–75% HRmax) between intervals

---

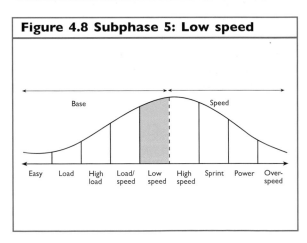

Figure 4.8 Subphase 5: Low speed

Table 4.5(a)	Training week in subphase 5 (triathlon/duathlon/multisport)						
Mon	Tues	Wed	Thurs	Fri	Sat	Sun
S/K (H)		S/K (S)		DAY OFF	S/K (L)	
	B (S)		B (H)			B (L)
R (H)		R (L)			**R (S)**	

Table 4.5(b)	Training week in subphase 5 (cycling/mountain biking/running/rowing)						
Mon	Tues	Wed	Thurs	Fri	Sat	Sun
E	S/H2	E	ML	DAY OFF	S/H1	L

The **bold** workouts are the training sessions where low speed training would be applied. The 1 and 2 show where low speed training should be emphasised first and second.

Period: Speed. Subphase 6: High speed

Anaerobic threshold is defined as the highest intensity that an athlete can maintain for approximately one hour. This equates to about a 40 km time trial pace on your bike or 16 km run pace. Anaerobic threshold training can be conducted as time trials or as less psychologically demanding intervals (e.g. 5–10 minutes). It improves your anaerobic threshold pace, thereby improving your race pace or your high steady state race pace. This subphase would occur one to two times per week and would last two to eight weeks (generally four).

Subphase 6: High speed

Specifics: Short intervals (16 km run or 40 km bike time trial pace). You should feel like you are 'hammering'

Effort: Difficult to converse (75–85% effort)

Sports:

    Swim: 250–500 m intervals

    Bike: 5–8 min intervals

    Run: 5 min intervals

    Kayak: 5–8 min intervals

    Row: 5–8 min intervals

Training heart rate: Anaerobic threshold rate (85–95% HRmax) for intervals; long slow distance rate (60–75% HRmax) between intervals

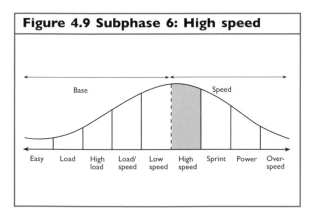

Figure 4.9 Subphase 6: High speed

Table 4.6(a)	Training week in subphase 6 (triathlon/duathlon/multisport					
Mon	Tues	Wed	Thurs	Fri	Sat	Sun
S/K (H)		S/K (S)		DAY OFF	S/K (L)	
	B (S)		B (H)			B (L)
R (H)		R (L)			R (S)	

Table 4.6(b)	Training week in subphase 6 (cycling/mountain biking/ running/rowing)					
Mon	Tues	Wed	Thurs	Fri	Sat	Sun
E	S/H2	E	ML	DAY OFF	S/H1	L

The **bold** workouts are the training sessions where high speed training would be applied. The 1 and 2 show where high speed should be emphasised first and second.

Subphases 7–9: Sprints, power, overspeed

The subphases of sprints, power and overspeed are not always applicable to most endurance sports, but there are some exceptions. The exceptions are:

- Mountain biking, distance running (particularly 10–21 km events) and some multisports require extensive sprints;
- Rowing uses sprints and power, and road cycling uses sprints, power and overspeed.

Subphase 7: Sprints (extensive/intensive)

The sprints subphase involves different forms of anaerobic or sprint training. Extensive sprints (45 seconds to 4 minutes) are used to improve sustained sprint speed at the start or end of a race, to bridge gaps, to break away from the peleton (pack) close to the finish, and to initiate breakaways. Intensive sprints (usually 10 seconds to 1 minute) are used to improve top sprinting speed. Intensive sprints can be broken down to uphill (50 m), crest (20–30 m uphill/ 20–30 m over the top) and flat (200–400 m) for running and cycling.

(Incidentally, uphill sprints occur during the load and high load subphases, crest sprints occur in the load/speed subphase and flat sprints occur in the speed phase.) Extensive and intensive sprint training occurs one to two times per week over one to four weeks (generally one to two)

Subphase 7: Sprints (extensive/intensive)

Specifics: Extensive sprints (long sprints) are 45 sec to 4 min sprints. Intensive sprints (short sprints) are 10 sec to 1 min sprints.

Effort: Very difficult to talk (90–100% effort)

Sports:

Swim: 100–400 m sprints
Bike: 200–4000 m sprints
Run: 100–1000 m sprints
Kayak: 100–500 m sprints
Row: 100–700 m sprints

Training heart rate: Not applicable

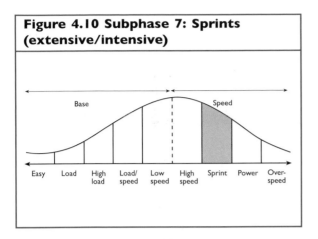

Figure 4.10 Subphase 7: Sprints (extensive/intensive)

Table 4.7(a)	Training week in subphase 7 (multisport)						
Mon	Tues	Wed	Thurs	Fri	Sat	Sun
K (H)		**K** (S)		DAY OFF	K (L)	
	B (S)		B (H)			B (L)
R (H)		R (L)			**R** (S)	

Table 4.7(b)	Training week in subphase 7 (cycling/mountain biking/ running/rowing)						
Mon	Tues	Wed	Thurs	Fri	Sat	Sun
E	S/H2	E	ML	DAY OFF	S/H1	L

The **bold** workouts are the training session where sprint training would be applied. The 1 and 2 show where sprint training should be emphasised first and second.

Subphase 8: Power (acceleration)

In cycling, power training is used to improve your ability to attack or 'jump' a rider, or the peleton. Power training can be conducted using plyometrics, by big gear wind-outs or by using a dip in the road to gain speed down a hill in a big gear, and then sprinting in the same gear up a short climb on the other side of the dip, stopping when you are not 'on top of the gear'.

Power training for rowing usually involves weight training, but may also involve power training in the boat.

You should feel strong during power training (i.e. you should not struggle to turn a gear over). The power subphase can occur one to two times per week over one to four weeks (generally one to two).

Subphase 8: Power (acceleration)

Specifics: Explosive acceleration
Effort: 100% effort
Training heart rate: Not applicable

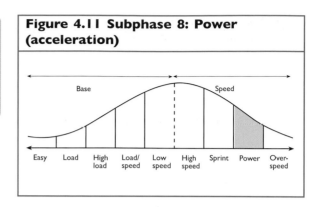

Figure 4.11 Subphase 8: Power (acceleration)

Table 4.8	Training week in subphase 8 (cycling/rowing)					
Mon	Tues	Wed	Thurs	Fri	Sat	Sun
E	S/H2	E	ML	DAY OFF	S/H1	L

The **bold** workouts are the training sessions where power training would be applied. The 1 and 2 show where power training should be emphasised first and second.

Subphase 9: Overspeed

Overspeed training involves increasing muscular contraction speed. It is the final aspect of speed-work. In cycling, downhill spinning sprints (sprinting downhill in a small gear at a high cadence) and motor pacing (high cadence drafting behind a vehicle to decrease the effects of wind resistance) are useful forms of overspeed.

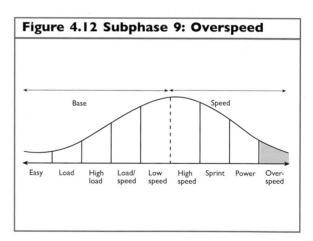

Figure 4.12 Subphase 9: Overspeed

Subphase 9: Overspeed

Specifics: Short downhill sprint intervals or motor pacing (drafting behind a motor vehicle) at above race pace speed to enhance muscle contraction speed
Effort: Moderate/low load and high speed
Reps: 100–200 m downhill, 120–200 rpm
Continuous effort: 5–100 km drafting behind a motor vehicle

Table 4.9	Training week in subphase 9 (cycling)						
Mon	Tues	Wed	Thurs	Fri	Sat	Sat	Sun
E	S/H2	E	ML	DAY OFF	S/H1	L

The **bold** workouts are the training sessions where overspeed training would be applied. The numbers 1 and 2 show where overspeed should be emphasised first and second.

Intensities and subphases – a piece of cake

In most cases, once you start to use a training intensity you continue to use it (to varying degrees) right up until race day. Each training intensity is slowly introduced and progressively increased over one to four weeks prior to the time when you begin to focus on the specific training subphase. Once a subphase reaches its peak emphasis, it is then maintained as other training subphases are initiated. Training subphases 1–5 (preparation, load, high load, load/speed, low speed) are introduced, focused on, and then maintained in progressively smaller amounts throughout the build-up. Sport-specific strength training must not be underrated. This must be maintained all the way through the programme.

Your body operates on a 'use it or lose it' principle. You train for a while and you perform better; you stop for a while and you perform worse. It takes a lot of work to build performance but surprisingly little to maintain it (20–30% of your biggest training volumes to hold most of your performance for 4 to 8 weeks). It's like building a house: it takes a lot of work to build but not nearly as much to maintain.

So when you start a build-up, you emphasise each form of training as you move through and then maintain it – you don't stop doing it. After you have done your first build-up, you maintain everything all of the time.

In other words, you might start with doing a little bit of load/speed subphase training very early on in the programme but will not emphasise this till you reach the load speed subphase where the training volume goes to maximum for this type of training. As you move into the next subphase the volume of that type of training is again reduced and maintained through until the end of the programme.

So, there it is. Those are all the ingredients needed for a good training recipe. But remember, training is a bit like baking a cake – it's not the ingredients that make a good cake, it's the way the chef puts them together.

To help you do this, an experienced athlete or coach could be called upon to advise you. They can use their experience to take the guesswork out of your training – this will save you learning the hard way!

Timing of subphases

When determining the timing of training subphases, you or your coach need to assess the racing intensity/pace for the competition you are aiming at. For example, if you are doing a long or ultra distance event (e.g. Ironman, marathon), race pace will be at approximately up-tempo training intensity.

For these events, up-tempo training occurs in the low speed subphase, i.e. at the start of speedwork, when race pace training always

Figure 4.13 Subphases in a cycling training programme

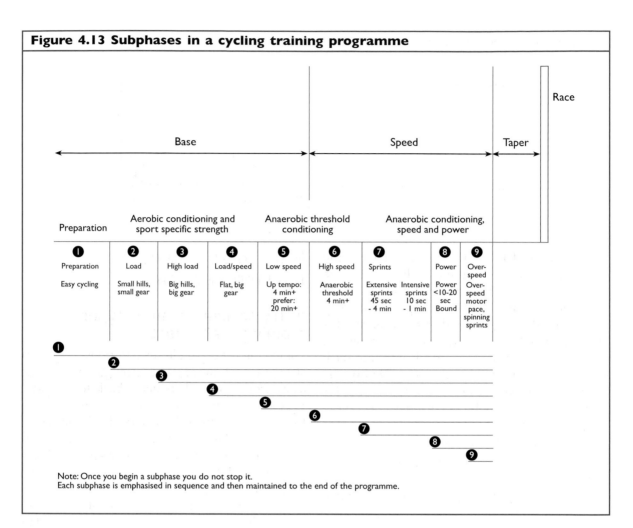

Base   Speed   Taper   Race

Preparation	Aerobic conditioning and sport specific strength			Anaerobic threshold conditioning		Anaerobic conditioning, speed and power		
❶	❷	❸	❹	❺	❻	❼	❽	❾
Preparation	Load	High load	Load/speed	Low speed	High speed	Sprints	Power	Over-speed
Easy cycling	Small hills, small gear	Big hills, big gear	Flat, big gear	Up tempo: 4 min+ prefer: 20 min+	Anaerobic threshold 4 min+	Extensive sprints 45 sec - 4 min / Intensive sprints 10 sec - 1 min	Power <10-20 sec Bound	Over-speed motor pace, spinning sprints

Note: Once you begin a subphase you do not stop it.
Each subphase is emphasised in sequence and then maintained to the end of the programme.

Figure 4.14 Subphase timing for a long-distance event

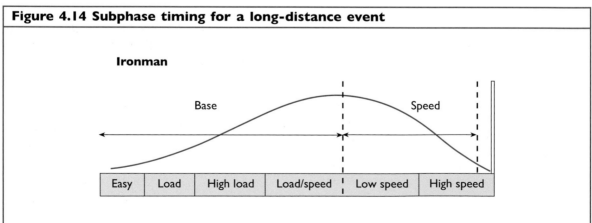

Ironman

Base   Speed

Easy	Load	High load	Load/speed	Low speed	High speed

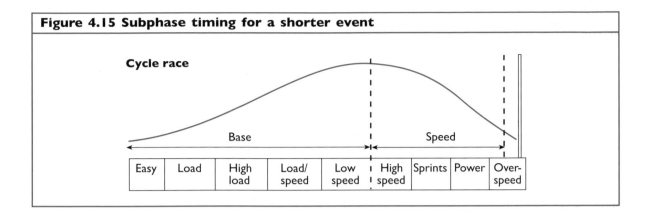

Figure 4.15 Subphase timing for a shorter event

Cycle race

Base — Speed

| Easy | Load | High load | Load/ speed | Low speed | High speed | Sprints | Power | Over- speed |

begins (*see* fig. 4.14). However, if you are doing a standard distance triathlon or 10 km run, the race pace will be closer to anaerobic threshold training intensity. This race pace intensity occurs in the high speed subphase, so this subphase would occur at the start of speedwork. This would push the low speed subphase back into base training (*see* fig. 4.15). Finally, be specific about what you require in training for your event. You might not need to use every subphase because:

- you might not have enough time;
- you might not require some of the intensities;
- you might want to spend more time on a specific subphase if you have a particular weakness.

How to use subphases

In the programmes in Part 3, there is a row for the subphase that is appropriate to the workout. For instance, in the cycling programme on page 267, Tuesday's workout in week 12 is 2. This tells the cyclist to focus on load i.e. with the main emphasis of the ride being hill training. Each subphase involves a different aspect of training.

How to structure a training session

1 Try to keep similar types of training well apart

For example, keep endurance sessions away from strength endurance, and strength endurance away from speed. This harks back to the principle of microcyclic training (*see* chapter 2, 'Day to day: microcycles'), where 'like' modes of training are kept as far apart from each other within the training week as possible. This helps recovery and therefore the absorption of training (very important!).

There are, of course, some situations where you might deliberately combine similar training modes (e.g. for triathlon: strength endurance hills on the bike followed by speed on the run to get used to running tired), but these situations are infrequent.

2 Train in the right order

If doing more than one type of training in the same workout, use the order set out in table 4.10 (cycling example):

The reason for training in this order is that you must be 'freshest' in order to do technique

Table 4.10	Correct order of training session (cycling)
Training type	Time
Warm-up	10 min
Technique	20 min
Speed	sprints 2 × 1 min (10 min rest between reps)
Speed	up-tempo and anaerobic threshold 3 × 5 min (5 min rest between reps)
Strength endurance	20 min, flat, big gear
Endurance	60 min endurance
Warm-down	10 min
Total time	172 min

Note: These forms of training would not normally be combined in one session!

work correctly and train at the higher intensities. This order not only applies in a workout but also in terms of prioritising recovery between workouts – speed and technique training require the longest recovery time, whereas endurance training requires the least. Here are two examples (table 4.11(a):incorrect; table 4.11(b): correct) of day-to-day scheduling that includes a speed training session:

Training Monday night and Tuesday morning leaves too little recovery time before the speed session.

By training Monday morning and leaving the speed session until Tuesday night, adequate recovery time is scheduled. Once again, there are exceptions to the rule (e.g. learning to do speedwork when tired) but in most cases this is the best format.

Table 4.11(a)	Example of incorrect day-to-day scheduling of training		
	Mon	Tues	Wed
a.m.	–	speed	endurance
p.m.	endurance	–	–

Table 4.11(b)	Example of correct day-to-day scheduling of training		
	Mon	Tues	Wed
a.m.	endurance	–	endurance
p.m.	–	speed	–

MANIPULATION OF TRAINING PRINCIPLES

5

Now that you understand the training principles for endurance events, it is time to start looking at how those principles can be manipulated to get different training effects. It is also time to look at how you can customise your programme to suit your racing and training commitments.

Strategies for continued improvement

As you start to train, you will see a big initial improvement, which is great for motivation. However, as time goes on you won't see the same level of improvement: you will therefore need to develop new training strategies in order to continue to progress and keep your interest levels up. In other words, you need to constantly manipulate and develop your training programme. The 'Big Picture' is that there are four key strategies you can use through your training career (4 – 16yrs) to achieve this.

Key strategy 1: the 'more is better' formula

When you first start training, it is likely that you use the 'more is better' approach – the more you train, the better you perform. This may well work fantastically for several years; however, at some stage you will find that performance increases won't come as easily

as they used to for the amount of time and effort you put in – you do more and more for less and less. This is known as 'the law of diminishing returns' (*see* page 31) and can be incredibly frustrating. It usually takes about two years of dedicated effort to end up here. A lot of athletes continue to do more and more and end up overtraining to a large extent. At this point, some athletes give up, while others look at what they can do differently. Overall, about 80 per cent of the athletic population adopts this 'more is better' approach.

Key strategy 2: the 'long and strong' formula

Some athletes discover that adding more resistance training to their programme, for example including more hill training, leads to the return of the big improvements of their earlier years. This is due to the fact that in most endurance events it is the leg muscles that suffer before the lungs: by the end of a race, you won't be gasping for breath, but your legs will be unable to carry on pushing hard. This means that strength endurance workouts will produce the most significant performance gains for the time spent training. However, this doesn't mean that you should do strength endurance only. You should still include endurance and speed training, but should emphasise strength endurance in each build-up phase at this stage in your sporting career. Most athletes reach this stage of training two-years after they begin training.

Unfortunately, at some stage you will once again hit a brick wall and stop seeing continued improvement, despite your effort. About 10 per cent of athletes encounter these problems, although a lot miss this stage and moved straight to key strategy 3.

Key strategy 3: the 'go harder' formula

At this stage, intensity and speed are key. The correct intensities, timing and number of workouts are crucial, otherwise you can wear yourself out.

On average, it takes four to five years to reach this point. One of the major mistakes that many athletes make is to move straight from volume ('more is better') to intensity ('go harder'), missing out the crucial element of strength endurance. Speed will allow you to go fast, but only for a short distance. Without strength endurance, speed is virtually useless in endurance events. However, as with previous stages, at some point you will once again become subject to the law of diminishing returns.

Key strategy 4: the 'smart training' formula

By this stage, you've emphasised all of the different types of training and now need to become smarter about what you do in order to get the most out of your training. In other words, you need to work out how to get the most return for the time spent, and how to train in the best, fastest and most effective way. After all, anyone can do huge amounts of hard training, but only the best know where to concentrate most of their efforts and what to drop out. The key is to try to find out what

works and to start to build your personal training formula as you go through your sporting career.

To summarise, improvement involves moving through a series of different training strategies over a period of years (*see* fig. 5.1). Each is important at different times, and missing any of them out will hinder your long-term potential. The trick is to see when you need to change and begin to move to the new strategy without getting bogged down or stuck on the old methods. Now we need to take a slightly smaller view and look at how training is set up through a year.

Length of seasons

In-season (generally eight to twelve weeks)

The timing and length of the competitive season varies according to how competition is structured and what your goals are. Some sports have a single peak in a year, for example national or world champs, where it is vital you peak on race day. In such cases, the in-season lasts only the day of the race (talk about pressure!). Other sports have a series of races, such as national series, best athlete over a series. In this case, the in-season can last several months.

The in-season generally lasts eight to twelve weeks with the athlete holding a 90 per cent plus performance level during that time. A 100 per cent performance level can only be maintained for approximately two to 14 days; this can occur one to three times during the in-season for most athletes. When an in-season lasts longer than 10 weeks, the athlete will need to repeat some aspects of pre-season training.

Figure 5.1 The life cycle of training

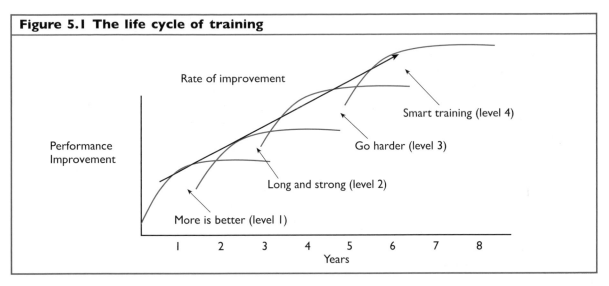

Pre-season (generally twelve to sixteen weeks)

The length of the pre-season depends somewhat on how long the race is. A long pre-season is required for long races (Ironman), while short races (10 km, cycle criterium) require a shorter pre-season. Training for a race series is highly variable and depends on your training history, the length of the series and the length of each race. Why does the pre-season vary in length? Simply because it will take you longer to reach the peak training mileages necessary for longer races (marathon, Half-Ironman), than for a shorter race (10 km, sprint triathlon). Remember that pre-season is made up of a base (two to six months) and a speed phase (four to eight weeks).

Off-season (generally four to sixteen weeks)

There is no problem with having a long off-season (although longer than six months is not advisable), as long as you maintain an active recovery programme, i.e. light, low-intensity activity. Four to twelve weeks is reasonable, less than four weeks is not advised. Elite athletes may have four

to eight weeks whereas novices will have eight to sixteen. Too short an off-season can tempt disaster because you may not recover completely before you begin your next base phase. This may lead to . . . you guessed it, overtraining!

Single versus double periodisation

If an athlete's peak races fall in the same season they will only need a single training periodisation (*see* fig. 5.2). However, international athletes often have a different seasonal make-up to their year with multiple seasons, for example competitions in both the northern and southern hemispheres, or in the case of a runner, a marathon in spring and autumn. This may result in a year looking like this:

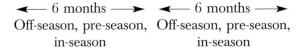

This type of double periodisation is illustrated in figure 5.3. In such cases, training periods are compressed, including off-seasons, though this needs to be carefully monitored as short off-seasons may increase the risk of burn-out. Note, though, that the more races you aim to peak for, the less chance you have of getting it right each time. International athletes with four or more peaks a season have to work very hard and very intelligently to peak precisely at the right time every time.

Length of training periods

Training periodisation (Base 1, Base 2, speed, taper) varies according to a number of variables. These are:

- Experience (how long you have been competing in the sport, your training history)
- Your ability and training tolerance
- Your age
- The length of the race you are training for

Experience has a big effect on training. If you have been involved in your sport for years, you can train harder and longer than if you are new to it. Tied up with this is age – up to a point, older athletes tend to be able to tolerate higher training volumes (one of the few advantages of getting older!).

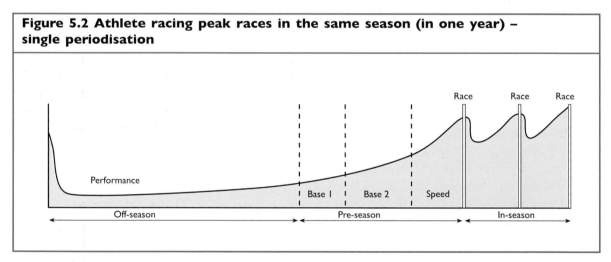

Figure 5.2 Athlete racing peak races in the same season (in one year) – single periodisation

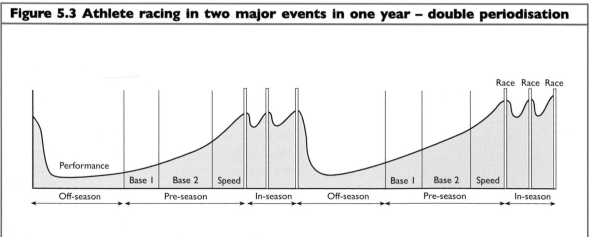

Figure 5.3 Athlete racing in two major events in one year – double periodisation

Ability also affects training. Some people are better suited to some sports than others; we have all seen those 'naturals' who perform well with relatively little preparation. These 'thoroughbreds' tend to be able to get away with less training than the rest of us. Of course, the history of sport is littered with examples of hard workers beating 'naturals'. Moral: it's hard to beat a good intelligent work ethic! Some athletes may also be able to naturally cope with greater training volumes and workloads than others.

The length of the race also determines the length of the training periods. As mentioned previously, longer races require higher mileages in training, and it takes time to build up to high mileages.

Let's look at the lengths of each of the training periods in turn.

Base 1

Base 1 can last between zero and eight weeks, depending on the number of problems that require work. If you have no real problems, Base 1 can be eliminated. But if there is a lot of work to be done, then Base 1 will probably last eight weeks. If you have a major injury problem to overcome, Base 1 can last for months.

Base 2

The length of Base 2 (eight to sixteen weeks) is primarily determined by the length of the race: the longer the race, the longer this phase needs to be to reach the required training mileages. To a lesser extent, Base 2 length is also determined by experience, age and ability. The younger or less experienced the athlete, the shorter the phases (Base 1, Base 2, speed) they can cope with.

Speed

This phase (four to eight weeks) is also determined by your experience, age and ability. Once again, younger and less experienced athletes will have a shorter phase (four weeks). More experienced athletes will cope with a longer speed phase (eight weeks). The length of the race (for sports dealt with in this book) has only a marginal effect on the length of the speedwork phase. This is because endurance events, unlike shorter races and sprint-oriented sports, don't require as great an emphasis on speed. Endurance events aren't called endurance events for nothing!

Taper

The length of the taper (two to 14 days) is again determined by the length of the race. The longer the race, the greater the training volume required, the greater the cumulative fatigue, and therefore the longer the taper. Taper is also affected by your recovery rate: the better you recover, the shorter the taper.

Variations in build-up time

What happens if you have more time than you need in build-up? Or not enough? In such situations (not uncommon, especially the latter), a programme may require major surgery.

Too much time

Having too much time is the better of the two problems to have. Generally, this means you can relax a little and start your build-up very gradually. You will also be able to concentrate on any small problems (flexibility, strength imbalances, niggling injuries) that may affect performance. Technique can also be emphasised for a while. Don't get sucked into building your training up too soon. The key is to build up *gradually*. With a long, gradual build-up, intermediate races should be done to help you maintain your enthusiasm, as well as help condition you for the major race or races ahead.

In cases where there is plenty of time, base training can be lengthened and one to two mini peaks can be scheduled into the programme. If you have more than six months until the start of your peak race build-up, you may want to focus on some similar events to help build your proficiency in the sport. For instance, if a build-up for Ironman takes about four months, and you have seven months, it would be useful to do a marathon or a long bike race in the three months before you begin your full Ironman build-up (*see* fig. 5.4). This will all add to your experience and performance.

If you have between three and six months until your peak race build-up begins, the 'more than six months' formula applies, except you would have only one mini peak involving a similar event. If you have less time than this, concentrate on slowly building up training and addressing specific problems.

Not enough time

If the time left until the race you want to aim at is too short for a complete build up, your programme will need to be compressed. This is a difficult and undesirable situation that long-term planning usually gets around. However, injuries, illness and the importance of an event (for example, an Olympic Games), sometimes mean you have to make the best of a bad situation. Nevertheless, if you have missed more than one-third to a half of your build-up, you should probably look at another event.

If you have lost less than one-third to a half of your build-up, the compression of your programme depends on the type of race you are facing and your previous background and experience. If it is a long race, the speed phase should be compressed or eliminated. If it is a short race, you will need to compress the base phase mainly, or compress slightly both the base and speed phases. Remember, though, that you need to do enough base work so you don't become overtrained or injured by speedwork.

How to manage training during the 'in-season'

Generally, you have two choices in peaking for races:

1 Spacing – peaks are spaced approximately six to eight weeks apart

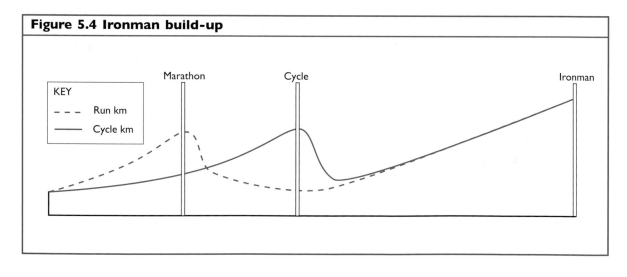

Figure 5.4 Ironman build-up

KEY
- - - Run km
—— Cycle km

Marathon Cycle Ironman

2 Clumping – peaks are clumped together over two to three weeks

The following outlines what to do for peak races at various periods.

Peak races two weeks apart

- less than two hour race – two weeks speed
- two to four hour race – two weeks speed
- longer than four hour race – two weeks speed

Four weeks apart

- less than two hour race – one week base/some speed; three weeks speed
- two to four hour race – two weeks base/some speed; two weeks speed
- longer than four hour race – three weeks base/some speed; one week speed

Six weeks apart

- less than one hour race – two weeks base/some speed; four weeks speed
- two to four hour race – three weeks base/some speed; three weeks speed
- longer than four hour race – four weeks base/some speed; two weeks speed

Ten weeks apart

- less than one hour race – four weeks base/two weeks some speed; four weeks speed
- two to four hour race – four weeks base/two weeks some speed; four weeks speed
- longer than four hour race – six weeks base/one week some speed; three weeks speed

Fifteen weeks apart

Do another pre-season build-up, possibly with a small off-season.

Mileage determination and peak mileage

'How many miles are you doing?' When one athlete wants to find out how much or how 'hard' another athlete is training, this is usually the question they ask. The question implies that more is better – which it very rarely is. Training is a dynamic process of which weekly mileage is just one ever-changing part, and often the least important part. Nevertheless, there is one week when you do need to count the miles in order to establish what your training volume will be in build-up. 'Peak-mileage week' is the highest training volume week in a training build-up.

Peak-mileage week placement in a build-up depends on the length of the race and, therefore, on whether distance or speed is the main training requirement. For a long race, peak mileages will occur closer to the race as mileage or distance is the main requirement (doing too much speedwork will stop you doing the mileage you need to do). For a cycle road race or tour, Ironman or marathon, the peak-mileage week will occur approximately three to five weeks before the event. For a short race, peak mileage is done further away from the race as speed receives a greater emphasis (too much mileage close to the race won't let you do the speedwork you need to do). For shorter races (standard distance triathlon or duathlon, rowing, most mountain bike races), peak mileage will be done six to ten weeks before the event.

Mileage increase

A common mistake is to increase your training mileage too quickly. In the first four to six weeks, a 5 to 10 per cent increase per week is sufficient, for example from 50 km to 55 km, or six hours to six hours 36 minutes. This doesn't seem like much, but it soon adds up over the weeks and months. After this, 10 per cent increases are okay while mileage is still fairly low. Finally, as you get close to peak mileage, 5 to 10 per cent increases are again acceptable.

Table 5.1	Peak mileage workouts for long races		
Sport		Race length	Approx. longest workout
Running	Marathon	42 km	30–36 km
	Half-marathon	21 km	21–26 km
	10 km	10 km	16–21 km
Sprint triathlon	Swim	700 m	700–2,000 m
	Bike	20 km	20–80 km
	Run	5 km	5–16 km
Olympic triathlon	Swim	1.5 km	1.5–3 km
	Bike	40 km	40–120 km
	Run	10 km	10–21 km
Half-Ironman	Swim	2 km	2–3.5 km
	Bike	90 km	90–140 km
	Run	21 km	21–26 km
Ironman	Swim	3.8 km	3.8–4.5 km
	Bike	180 km	160–200 km
	Run	42 km	26–36 km
Mountain biking	Standard race	2–3 hr	3.5–4.5 hr
Cycling	40 km	40 km	80–120 km
	80 km	80 km	80–140 km
	160 km	160 km	160–200 km
	Tour	700–1,100 km	160–200 km
Rowing	Standard race	2,000 m	15,000–25,000 m
Duathlon, short	Run	5 km x 2	16–21 km
	Bike	40 km	40–120 km
Duathlon, long	Run	10 km x 2	20–26 km
	Bike	60 km	60–120 km

Multisport – depends on race.
Run: up to duration or add 40–60% to race length for sub-3-hour races
Bike and kayak: up to race distance or add 40–60% to race length for sub-3-hour races

First, though, you need to work out when you want your peak-mileage week to occur. You can then work out the weekly mileages for your build-up, working back from the peak-mileage week. The way to do this is explained, step-by-step, in chapter 7.

Peak-mileage workouts (that is, the longest workout you will do in training for a particular event) vary depending on the length of the race and the sport you are training in. In general, for longer races, athletes tend not to train up to the full race distance (as this can be too taxing, unless they are training in a low-impact/stress sport), whereas shorter races often involve overdistance training (workouts longer than the race distance). High-impact/stress sports, such as running, are less likely to involve training up to full race distance for longer races than low-impact/stress sports such as cycling. Table 5.1 includes some examples of peak-mileage workouts.

Strength

If we were to define speed on a bike it would be like this:

$$Speed = cadence \times gear$$

In its simplest terms, if you can push a big gear and turn it over fast you have high speed. Not rocket science, but important just the same.

One of the key motivators for the formation of the Lydiard principles (taking someone's natural speed and building strength endurance then speed endurance) was a book that was written by F. A. M. Webster in the 1930s. While reading this book, Arthur Lydiard came across a statement written in a time when the mile world record was around 4:13. It said that the four-minute mile would be broken someday because the human body was *able* to go at the correct speed, it just could not *endure* the speed. Arthur noticed the word 'endure', and the great Lydiard endurance training principles were born.

In other words, being able to generate speed is one thing, but having the ability to endure the speed generated is another thing entirely. This leads to an adjustment in the equation cited above:

Ability to endure speed = ability to endure the cadence + ability to endure the gear

Or put more simply:

Speed endurance = cadence endurance + gear endurance

In order to work out the magic ingredient, look at table 5.2.

Look at the gear and pedalling frequency. The gear is shown by designating the chainring and the rear cog and then showing the 'rollout', which is the section of the table you should focus on. 'Rollout' is the distance in metres it takes for the gear to make one complete revolution (defined as the left pedal, starting from the top of the pedal stroke, rotating around once back to the top of pedal stroke). A small gear has a shorter 'rollout'; it might be six metres instead of eight metres. The bigger the gear you can push, the stronger you are. The pedalling frequency or cadence is the number of times the gear is turned over per minute. A pedalling frequency of 100 indicates that the left pedal has turned over 100 complete revolutions in a minute.

What table 5.2 therefore shows us is that, in the successful attempts to break the world cycling 1-hour record from 1937 to the present day, pedal cadence has remained the same; the

Table 5.2	Gear and pedalling frequency for the world hour record					
YEAR	NAME	PLACE	GAIN (m)	DIST (m)	GEAR	FREQUENCY
1937	Slaats (NL)	Milan	160	45,535	24 × 7 = 7.32	103.6
1937	Archambaud (Fr)	Milan	280	45,817	24 × 7 = 7.32	104.3
1942	Coppi (It)	Milan	31	45, 848	52 × 15 = 7.4	103.3
1956	Anquetil (Fr)	Milan	311	46, 159	52 × 15 = 7.4	103.9
1956	Baldini (Fr)	Milan	234	46, 393	52 × 15 = 7.4	104.4
1957	Riviere (Fr)	Milan	530	46, 923	52 × 15 = 7.4	105.7
1958	Riviere (Fr)	Milan	423	47, 346	53 × 15 = 7.54	104.6
1967	Bracke (Bel)	Rome	747	48, 093	53 × 15 = 7.54	106.3
1968	Ritter (Den)	Mexico City	560	48, 653	54 × 15 = 7.69	105.4
1972	Merckx (Bel)	Mexico City	778	49, 431	52 × 14 = 7.93	103.9
1984	Mosser (It)	Mexico City	1,377	50, 808	56 × 15 = 8.17	103.6
1984	Mosser (It)	Mexico City	343	51, 151	57 × 15 = 8.27	103
1993	Obree (GB)	Hamar	445	51, 596	52 × 12 = 9.25	92.9
1993	Boardman (GB)	Bordeaux	674	52, 570	53 × 13 = 8.70	100.1
1994	Obree (GB)	Bordeaux	443	52, 713	52 × 12 = 9.25	94.9
1994	Indurain (Sp)	Bordeaux	327	53, 040	59 × 14 = 8.86	100.9
1994	Romiger (Swi)	Bordeaux	792	53, 832	59 × 14 = 8.86	101.3
1994	Romiger (Swi)	Bordeaux	1,459	55, 291	60 × 14 = 9.02	102.2
1996	Boardman (GB)	Manchester	1,084	56, 375	56 × 13 = 9.02	104.2

only real change is in the size of the gear. Therefore, the limiting factor is the size of the gear. This can be applied to other sports: in running it is stride length, in swimming it is distance per stroke, and so on.

Going back to the equation, we can see where the weak point is in most cases: gear endurance. Therefore, increasing the resistance in our training without injuring ourselves, and getting used to pushing higher resistances for longer, is an important aspect of increasing speed. We talk about training for an endurance event, but in fact we are training for a strength endurance event.

Types of speedwork

Speed training is required to some degree for most racing situations. It increases your competitive capabilities by simulating race conditions and intensities, and this helps you adapt physically and psychologically to the demands of racing. Speedwork can be performed at various intensities, but it needs to be specific to your racing needs – going flat out may feel good, but it won't help your performance if you don't need to race flat out!

Speedwork during training will generally move from short distances with long rests at the start of speedwork, to longer distances with shorter rests at the end. This allows you to develop your tolerance to speedwork gradually. Without this gradual approach you are likely to become overtired and you will not achieve the desired training response. Submaximal work improves your steady state speed.

Sprint or anaerobic speedwork generally follows a slightly different format. Progression here is from longer sprints (for speed endurance development) to shorter sprints (for top speed, power and acceleration development). Rest periods between sprint intervals vary from very short (to improve sprint recovery or recovery from oxygen debt) to long (between maximal sprint efforts). Variations in sprint training depend on the sport or on the requirements of particular races – you can emphasise speed endurance, top speed or acceleration/power as you need to. Common forms of speedwork for endurance athletes are racing, intervals, time trials and sprints.

	Time trials	Time trials
Intervals →	Intervals (if no →	Intervals
	specific races)	Sprints (if needed)
	Races	Races

Tables 5.3 and 5.4 summarise the types of submaximal and high-intensity training for speedwork as discussed in chapters 3 and 4. Details on types of low-intensity training are also included.

Table 5.3	Types of speedwork and their use in each sport						
Training type	Effort (approx.)	Duration (approx.)	Tri/multi	Run	Cycle	Mountain bike	Row
Power	100%	<10–20 sec	–	–	Jumps	–	Stroke
Intensive sprints	100%	10 sec–1 min	–	–	Jumps, bridge gaps, final sprints	Accel	First and last 500 m
Extensive sprints	95–100%	45 sec–4 min	–	Leg speed, some starts	Bridge gaps, final sprints	Accel	First and last 500 m
Submaximal intervals	85–95%	>4 min	Approx. race pace	Approx. race pace	Peloton, riding, TTS, breaks	Approx. race pace	Approx. race pace

Key: Accel = acceleration; TTS = time trials; – = intensity not used.
Note: Low-intensity training (up-tempo, LSD and active recovery) are not classed as speedwork.

Table 5.4	Training intensities and their effort				
Training type	Duration (approx.)	Effort (approx.)	Subjective pace	Training effect	Interval example
Power	<10–20 sec	100%	V. intense, v. short	Improves initial accel.	V. short 10–15 sec then rest to recovery; plyometrics
Intensive sprints	10 sec–1 min	100%	V. intense, unable to converse	Improves max. explosive sprint	Short 30 sec–1 min then rest to recovery (in most cases)
Extensive sprints	45 sec–4 min	95–100%	Intense, very difficult to converse	Improves max. sustained sprint pace	Moderate 1–3 min; variable recovery
Submaximal intervals	>4 min	85–95%	Moderately intense, moderate to difficult to converse	Improves max. steady-state pace	Long intervals usually 4–20 min, or TTS; dec recovery
Up-tempo	>4 min	75–85%	Moderately easy to converse	Progressive intensity, inc bridge btwn LSD and speedwork	V. long intervals, progressive intensity inc and duration dec; rest to recovery
Long slow distance	>4 min	60–75%	Easy to converse	Inc training tolerance and inc ability to cope with dist; basic conditioning	Continuous
Active	>4 min	<60%	V. easy to converse	Assists recovery, no real training effect	Continuous

Key: Int = intervals; inc = increase; dec = decrease; dist = distance; LSD = long slow distance; accel = acceleration; TTS = time trials

Intervals (aerobic/anaerobic threshold)

Intervals are designed to increase gradually the amount of race pace stress on your body. Initially, you need to start your intervals off with short periods of work and long periods of rest. You will progress gradually to long periods of work and short periods of rest as you adapt to the increasing volume and the interval intensity. Eventually, you will train at race intensity for most, if not all, of the distance you are aiming to race over.

Heart rate monitors can be used to achieve not only the correct interval intensity, but also the correct rest periods between intervals. Correct interval intensity, as indicated by a heart rate monitor, is generally determined by laboratory testing. This can also be determined, although less accurately, by indirect calculations (*see* pages 36–37).

Most aerobic/anaerobic threshold intervals for endurance sports are performed at or near maximum steady state pace. Recovery between intervals can be set to a pre-selected time or the time it takes for your heart rate to drop to a specified level (e.g. 40 to 50 beats below interval exercise heart rate). The less fit you are the longer the recovery period because your heart rate will take longer to return to the specified level. Figure 5.5 gives an example of interval sessions used by a runner during a four-week training period.

Very short intervals with long rests should be used in your taper week before races. This will help you maintain race pace form, but avoid fatigue as race day approaches.

Time trials

Time trials involve long periods of continuous exertion close to race pace. They usually last 30 to 60 minutes for most sub-three-hour races. The only exception to that in this book is rowing. Rowing time trials last approximately three to seven minutes, because rowing races are over a relatively short distance (2000 m).

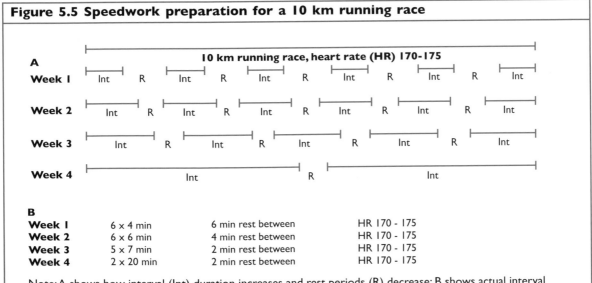

Figure 5.5 Speedwork preparation for a 10 km running race

B			
Week 1	6 x 4 min	6 min rest between	HR 170 - 175
Week 2	6 x 6 min	4 min rest between	HR 170 - 175
Week 3	5 x 7 min	2 min rest between	HR 170 - 175
Week 4	2 x 20 min	2 min rest between	HR 170 - 175

Note: A shows how interval (Int) duration increases and rest periods (R) decrease; B shows actual interval and rest duration, and interval heart rates (HR).

In essence, time trials are mini race simulations. They should start at very short distances and progress to longer distances. They can be very tiring and preferably should only be done late in the speedwork phase after intervals have already been done.

If there are no effective warm-up races available, then time trials are the next best thing. But remember that races and time trials are similar workouts and so both should not be done in the same week. Neither should time trials be done the week before or the week after a race. No more than one time trial should be done each week, and it is best only to do them every two to four weeks (elite, every one to two weeks; intermediate, every two to four weeks; novice, no time trials, just intervals).

Racing

Races are very much like time trials, but with the added bonus of competition. Races should preferably only be done towards the middle and latter stages of the speedwork phase after a period on intervals. Do not race every week unless it is necessary (e.g. a race series), or unless it has been built into your programme. Avoid speedwork two to four days before and after a race (*see* 'Tapering for races', page 86).

Sprints and sprint intervals (anaerobic)

Sprints are a type of high-intensity interval. They are used to develop your ability to cope with oxygen debt and to develop maximum pace. The difference between sprints and aerobic/anaerobic threshold intervals is that sprints are shorter and do not always require a reduction in the rest period.

Some sprints will have reduced rest periods, while others will have rests that allow full recovery as the sprint is designed to improve short distance speed and not sustained top speed.

The only so-called endurance sports that use sprint training are cycling (road and mountain biking) and rowing, although very short sprints or 'stride outs' may be used to develop leg speed for running. A speedwork session may look like this: 6 x 1 min at 100 per cent effort with a 2 min rest between efforts.

Other forms of speedwork

Another form of speedwork is 'fartlek' (a Swedish term meaning speedplay). Your interval/sprint lengths are varied in both duration/intensity and recovery time, based on how you feel.

Overspeed is used by cyclists and short distance runners to increase muscular contraction speed. This involves exercising at a slightly faster biomechanical pace than race pace.

'Dead leg' speedwork can also be used to get your body used to exercising on tired legs. This may involve hill training immediately followed by speedwork.

In general, doing speedwork in the afternoon is best. Your body seems to perform better then.

Use of speedwork

Determination of training intensities

When looking at your training requirements for a specific race, think about what training period you are in, and the intensity of the training you will need to do. In the base period, low-intensity training is required. During the speed phase, though, you will need to do some training at race pace and practise aspects of racing such as accelerating, extensive and intensive sprints, and hill climbing. This all helps to simulate race conditions. The questions you need ask yourself, therefore, are *which* training intensities, *when* and *how much*? Let's start with *which*.

If the race is going to involve some long or extended sprints, then you will need to do some high-intensity (HI) training incorporating extensive sprinting. This is the rule of specificity! You need to work out what intensities you should train at and when (*see* Part 3 Specific Sample Programmes for help). If you are doing speed phase training for a 40 km cycle criterium, for instance, mileage is not as important as speedwork. You would need to concentrate on high steady state speed (SM), sprinting/acceleration (HI; extensive, intensive and power), and cornering, as criteriums are generally on short, fast, tight courses.

If, on the other pedal, you were training for a 1400 km cycle tour over nine days, most of your training would consist of high mileage at low intensity (LO). After all, there is no point in being fast if you can't complete the tour. LO training would still be done in the speed phase to maintain base, but at low volume. Different sports also have different demands in terms of training intensities. Rowing, for example, requires greater volumes of high-intensity training than mountain biking. Ironman triathletes require greater training volumes at lower intensities than short-course triathletes. Now for the *when* part.

Different races and different courses in the same sport require slightly different approaches in terms of training intensities. Deciding which training intensities you will need to emphasise is only half the challenge. You have to decide *when* during the training period the different intensities need to occur. For example, SM starts in the speedwork phase, HI towards the middle to end of speedwork. Realise that your body has a good memory for duration/distance training (i.e. base). This means you can drop your training volumes to 50 to 70 per cent of peak volumes and your body will remember the long work you did for some time. On the other hand, your body has a lousy memory for speedwork. If you eliminate speedwork from your programme, you start to slow down virtually immediately (approximately four to fourteen days). So speedwork needs to be maintained until a few days before the race. Now, *how much*? Or to put it less succinctly, what proportion of the training is done at each intensity?

To work this out, you will also need to work out how much each intensity contributes to a race and then allocate training accordingly *during the speedwork phase*. For example, for elite marathoners, since a marathon is 99 per cent submaximal and below, no high-intensity training is necessary! If a race is short and hilly with a lot of sprinting, such as a cycle race, the main training requirement will be SM, with some HI work for the sprints, and LO work to maintain base. A lot of hill training would also be carried out. The hill training and the low-intensity work would occur mainly in the base phase, with submaximal and high-intensity work (including hill intervals and sprinting) happening in the speed phase. You can even assign percentages to each intensity. SM, extensive and intensive sprints, and power will only account for a maximum of 10 to 15 per cent of total mileage in the speed phase. The rest will be up-tempo, long slow distance (LSD) and active recovery.

In general, match your training intensities to those of the race. But remember that training generally progresses from long and slow to short and fast, relative to the race pace you are trying to achieve. And don't forget that if you need to do some high-intensity training during the speed phase, do some submaximal training first. The body does not like to jump from slow to fast in one leap.

Table 5.5 provides an example of how the final two to three weeks of base before speedwork starts might look like.

Table 5.5	Sample programme for final two to three weeks of base before speedwork					
Mon	Tues	Wed	Thurs	Fri	Sat	Sun
LO	UT	LO	UT	D/O	LO	LO (Long)

Key: LO = low-intensity; UT = up-tempo (intermediate intensity); D/O = day off.

Up-tempo days slowly progress from very slow training in the final weeks of the base period to speed training during the speed phase. This should be a careful progression. No sudden changes in training tempo should occur from week to week. Not only would a sudden tempo change increase the likelihood of injury, it might lead to you peaking too early, or training over-load in the last few weeks of the base phase. Up-tempo workouts should be done on the same days of the week you will later do your speed-work on. All other days are maintained at LO.

Tables 5.6(a) and (b) are examples of how base and speed phases might be set out for a road cyclist. They show that speed is introduced into the programme very gradually.

Week	Meso-cycle	Mon	Tues	Wed	Thurs	Fri	Sat	Sun	HR
1	H	28 kph Cont	LO	28 kph Cont	LO	D/O	LO	LO	135–140
2	H	28 kph Cont	LO	28 kph Cont	LO	D/O	LO	LO	135–140
3	E	28 kph Cont	LO	28 kph Cont	LO	D/O	LO	LO	135–140
4	H	28 kph Cont	LO	28 kph Cont	LO	D/O	LO	LO	135–140
5	H	28 kph Cont	LO	28 kph Cont	LO	D/O	LO	LO	135–140
6	E	28 kph Cont	LO	28 kph Cont	LO	D/O	LO	LO	135–140
7	H	32 kph Cont (UT)	LO	32 kph Cont (UT)	LO	D/O	LO	LO	145–150/ 140–145
8	H	32 kph Cont (UT)	LO	32 kph Cont (UT)	LO	D/O	LO	LO	145–150/ 140–145

Table 5.6(a) Road cyclist: base phase

Table 5.6(b)	Road cyclist: speed phase								
Week	Meso-cycle	Mon	Tues	Wed	Thurs	Fri	Sat	Sun	HR
1	E	LO	50% Ints* 38 kph	LO	LO	D/O	50% Ints* 38 kph	LO	165–170
2	H	LO	Ints* 39 kph	LO	LO	D/O	Ints* 39 kph	LO	170–175
3	H	LO	Ints* 40 kph	LO	LO	D/O	Ints* 40 kph	LO	175–180
4	E	LO	50% Ints* 40 kph	LO	LO	D/O	50% Ints* 40 kph	LO	175–180
5	H	LO 41 kph	Ints*	LO	LO	D/O 41 kph	Ints*	LO	180–185

Key: HR = Heart rates; H = hard week; E = easy week; kph = kilometres per hour; Cont = continuous; LO = low-intensity; UT = up-tempo; D/O = day off; Ints = intervals; 50% Ints = 50% number of usual intervals; * = submaximal intensity. Note: Speeds and heart rates are given as examples only to show increases in speed; these will vary from person to person; all low-intensity workouts are done at a heart rate of 135–140; 5–10 k on/10–15 k off; 5–10 k on/10–15 k off = up-tempo interval in the final two weeks (weeks 7 and 8) of base.

Mesocycles and speedwork

During the easy weeks of a mesocycle, training volume is reduced. The volume of speedwork is also reduced. The training intensity, however, is not reduced!

Table 5.7 provides an example of how this works in the speedwork phase.

Maximum number of speed days per week

In most single-discipline sports, for example rowing or running, speedwork can only be performed as a complete session a couple of times per week during the speed phase. All other workouts are done at a low intensity (tired athletes please note!) to maintain base. One exception is swimming, as it is less taxing on the body because the bodyweight is being supported. Indeed, some speedwork can be done every session in swimming. Generally, low-impact, high-fluidity sports allow more speedwork sessions per week, for example swimmers and cyclists can tolerate more speed-work than runners. In multidiscipline training, one speed session can occur in each discipline each week. However, more speed sessions can usually be done overall as the sessions are spread across a number of disciplines.

The amount of time you have been in the sport and your recovery rate also determine how many speedwork sessions you can handle during the speedwork phase. Table 5.8 provides some recommendations.

Peaking

> Correct training + correct timing = peaking

The key to top performance is being able to peak effectively. Most athletes, particularly inexperienced ones, tend to reach very good racing form, but do not peak fully. And there is a big difference between good form and peak form. (At a world champs that difference may mean finishing tenth instead of first!)

Base and speed phases, and warm-up races, are all deliberately set around a high-priority race or races so that you reach peak and perform at your best on the day or days that matter. Peaking encompasses all facets of training. Important points for peaking:

- Correct structure of programme
- Specificity of programme
- Applicability to athlete
- Elimination of training errors (too much, too little, too fast, too slow)
- Timing of the programme (too early, too late)
- Correct programme balance (work/rest, sport vs sport, workout requirement vs workout requirement, training frequency)

- Understand your training
- Analysis of training

If you take all these key points into account, you will achieve a peak performance on the right day. And as you get more experienced, your ability to peak will improve as you learn to refine your training.

Peak too early or too late, and you will race slow. Remember, a true peak brings all facets of training together at precisely one time. Most athletes manage to bring most facets together and some athletes none. By manipulating the principles above, you will be able to bring all facets of training together and maximise performance whenever you need to. Remember, peaking is rather like walking a tightrope – a matter of balance.

Time-saving tricks

Time-saving trick 1: Lots of little workouts beat several big workouts

Look at sample workout weeks A and B (tables 5.12(a) and (b).

Table 5.12(a)	Sample workout week A							
	Mon	Tues	Wed	Thurs	Fri	Sat	Sun	No. of workouts
Kayak (min)	20	30		20	60	120		5
Bike (min)		30	20	20		20	120	5
Run (min)	30		90	20		10	10	5
Total (min)	50	60	110	60	60	150	130	

Table 5.12(b)	Sample workout week B							
	Mon	Tues	Wed	Thurs	Fri	Sat	Sun	No. of workouts
Kayak (min)	30		20		60			3
Bike (min)		60		60		120	130	4
Run (min)	20		80			30		3
Total (min)	50	60	110	60	60	150	130	

The same amount of time is spent per day but example A has more workouts. While you should mix things up a little (for example, do two weeks of A for every week of B), A is still better on average. You may think it would be a waste of time putting on your running gear for 20 minutes, but just try it and you will see the difference. It seems that lots of little workouts keeps the body's motor warm, which seems to lead to better performance. Also, doing lots of big workouts leads to more wear and tear, so in most cases one or two larger workouts and then several of small workouts will make you less tired, fitter and faster.

Workouts generally fall into two camps: those that train you and those that maintain you. Those 10-minute 'keep the motor warm' workouts don't get you fitter, but they stop you from moving backwards and also keep you 'warm' and slightly fresher for the next big workout so you get more out of it.

Value of time saving trick over the year:
Zero, but probable performance increase.

Time-saving trick 2: short build-up blocks

12-week build-ups seem to work for most athletes, while top athletes and time-scarce athletes generally respond best on eight-week blocks. A busy person knows he can concentrate for 8 weeks solidly, but the longer you push that out the more things unravel. So, two 8-week blocks with a 2–3-week break in between is better than one long haul. If you have a lot of responsibilities, a heavy load at work and a family, your 'life load' will be high and you will have less energy that can be allocated to training. So, short blocks are better. A busy person on a long programme usually will get very flat, physically and mentally, and often gets chronic fatigue.

Value of time saving trick over the year:

A traditional training setup would look something like this:

3 x 12–16-week build-up blocks = 42 weeks training
3 x 3 weeks rest between = 9 weeks resting
Total = 51 weeks (add 1 more rest week to make 52)

The time-saving setup would look like this:

4 x 9-week build-up blocks = 36 weeks training
4 x 4 week rest between = 16 weeks resting
Total = 52 weeks

Total time saving is therefore 7 weeks of training (approximately 70 hours).

Time-saving trick 3: use alternate weeks

Your body can remember most forms of training for at least a few weeks. Keeping your body guessing can therefore enhance performance gains. Tables 5.13(a), (b) and (c) illustrate a training programme emphasising cycling in the first week, then focusing on running in the second week. Week 3 should be an easy week with a moderate swim emphasis.

Training in this way means that your body remembers the emphasised training in each week. If you combine the totals of the biggest swim week, (260 min), the big bike week (390 min) and the big run week (290 min), you would end up with a huge training week and most of the performance results that that would entail, without actually ever doing the big training week. Your maximum week would be 620 min, but you get close to the result of a 940-min training week. It's almost like you trick your

Table 5.13(a)	First hard week of mesocycle (2H, 1E): bike emphasis							
	Mon	Tues	Wed	Thurs	Fri	Sat	Sun	Total
Swim (min)	40		20		60	30		150
Bike (min)		60	50	60		40	180	390
Run (min)	20		40			20		80
Total (min)	60	60	110	60	60	90	180	620

Table 5.13(b)	Second hard week of mesocycle (2H, 1E): run emphasis							
	Mon	Tues	Wed	Thurs	Fri	Sat	Sun	Total
Swim (min)	30		20			30		80
Bike (min)		30		30			90	150
Run (min)	30	30	80	30		60	60	290
Total (min)	60	60	100	60	0	90	150	520

Table 5.13(c)	Easy week of mesocycle (2H, 1E): swim emphasis							
	Mon	Tues	Wed	Thurs	Fri	Sat	Sun	Total
Swim (min)	30	30	60	20		60	60	260
Bike (min)		30		40			60	130
Run (min)	30		40			30	60	160
Total (min)	60	60	100	60	0	90	180	550

body into thinking it did a big training week that you never actually do.

Alternate week training is not recommended for inexperienced athletes as the training volume jumps can be extreme. Therefore, it is only advised for athletes with a solid training history.

Value of time-saving trick over the year:

Build-up peak week totalling 620 min; effect using alternate weeks is close to doing 940 min. 940 min divided by 620 min = 35% time saved per build-up.
Let's say you do 171 hours of training per build-up. 35% of that is 60 hours.
4 build-ups per year at 60 hours is 240 hours total. Time saving for the year = 240 hours.

Time-saving trick 4: supercompensation weeks

Your body has two ways of training. One is known as 'progressive overload' where you do a bit of training, then recover, then do a bit more, then recover, and so on until you reach your training objectives. However, if we look at very long distance races like adventure races and some ultra races (running, cycling) for example, traditional 'progressive

overload' logic breaks down. You can't do a days racing, take time to recover, then do two days of racing, then recover, then do three days of racing, then recover, and so on up to for example 10 days and then go and do a big 'ultra race'. It doesn't work like that. Traditional training breaks down.

This is where the second type of training comes in: shock training, crash training or superovercompensation. This involves giving your body a bigger than usual shock or surprise and is based on the logic that the magnitude of the shock on the body (without producing illness or injury) is equal to the magnitude of response or gain in fitness, as long as you recover properly from it (*see* fig. 3.3). In other words, no shock or stimulus equals no response; big shock equals big reaction. So, you can use several big shock weeks and the rest of your training would be smaller volumes of traditional progressive overload. Shock weeks should occur three to seven weeks before the race, depending on its distance (shocks weeks were even used by the East Germans the week before a big race, but this has proved to be a little unpredictable). The downside is that shock weeks cost a lot of energy and can't be used very often maybe one or two times in the build-up. For example, for an Ironman you might do nine weeks with a 12- to 15-hour-maximum week of training, then have a week of shock training at around 25 to 30 hours.

Value of time saving trick over the year:

50 hours saved per buildup (171 hrs – 121 hrs = 50 hrs).

Time-saving over the year (4 x build-ups): 4 x 50 hrs = 200 hrs

Time-saving trick 5: simulation weeks/workouts/weekends

An event is defined as a series of tasks, specific to the course, performed one after the other in the correct sequence, allowing you to cover the course as quickly and efficiently as possible.

A simulation week, workout or weekend is where your training is as close to race conditions as possible. Most of the time you will not be doing the training at speed, but you almost definitely want to cover as many of the specific situations that you will encounter in the race as

possible. The ideal strategy is to perform simulations on the course you will race on. This is called leveraging your training.

Value of time-saving trick over the year:

Time saving is zero, but you will see higher performance gains for time spent. Also, because simulation weeks are more valuable than standard training you could reduce some of your other training if you wanted to.

Time-saving trick 6: the 80/20 rule

The 80/20 rule states that 80 per cent of your results come from 20 per cent of your workouts. Therefore, identifying the highest value workouts and doing them well is very important. Knowing which workouts you can and can't drop from your training also helps save time.

Value of time-saving trick over the year:

Time saving is zero but you will see higher performance gains for time spent.

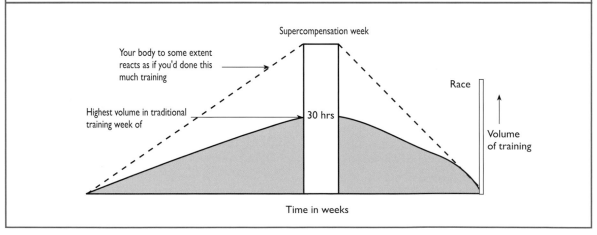

Figure 5.12 The benefits of a superovercompensation week: your body reacts as if you did progressive overload to get up to 30 hours per week without all the extra training

Time-saving trick 7: objectives

The clearer your goals and objectives are, the clearer the outcomes will be – and no objectives equals no planned outcome. Having a clear training objective for every workout allows you to get more out of your time and effort. Furthermore, the more objectives that you can clearly achieve per workout, the better the movement forward. Top athletes normally have three objectives per workout: a physical objective, for example training on the bike and doing big gear work; a technical objective, for example working on how technically well and fluidly they pedal; and a tactical objective, for example things that they need to practise thinking about for use in the race, such as taking the shortest line. Imagine if every time you went out the door you had three clear objectives. You might be able to increase your workout effectiveness by as much as 150 per cent. Imagine doing that workout to workout, week to week, month to month for a whole year.

Value of time-saving trick over the year:

Time saving is zero, but you will see higher performance gains for time spent.

Time-saving trick 8: emphasise

This means emphasising one sport at a time and only applies to multi-discipline sports. Rather than trying to work on everything at once, alternate sports in each training block or build-up over the year: *emphasise one sport while maintaining your other disciplines* in the build-up for eight weeks, then go into an off-season. When you move back into training for the next build-up, do the same with another sport for the next eight weeks. For example, a triathlete might choose to emphasise cycling three build-ups out from the race, then move to a running focus two build-ups out, and finally go to working on all sports evenly going into the final build-up before peaking for the key event (*see* fig. 5.13). This will lead to greater improvements. For this particular cyclist, who knows her specific strength and weaknesses and thus the areas she needs to focus on, this will lead to the greatest improvement.

You may also choose to emphasise a particular type of training in the build-up. For instance, you might emphasise strength over speed or endurance. If you try to emphasise strength, speed and endurance in every build up, the

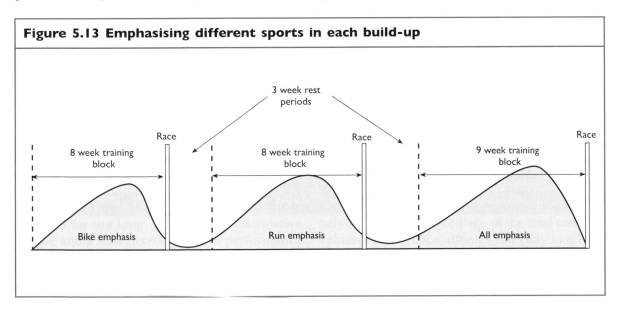

Figure 5.13 Emphasising different sports in each build-up

3 week rest periods

Race

Race

Race

8 week training block

8 week training block

9 week training block

Bike emphasis

Run emphasis

All emphasis

FUNDAMENTALS THAT AID TRAINING AND PERFORMANCE

6

Warming up and warming down

Warming up and warming down are an extremely important part of each workout.

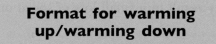

Format for warming up/warming down

warm-up ➔ stretch ➔ workout ➔ warm-down ➔ stretch

Warm-up

Warm-ups are aimed at gradually bringing the body up to the exercise pace/intensity level at which you will be training. For instance, a warm-up for intervals will involve a longer warm-up, gradually building to interval intensity, than a warm-up for a long slow distance workout. Warm-ups prepare you for exercise, reduce the chance of injury and increase the effectiveness of the workout (particularly for higher intensity workouts). The main goals of the warm-up are to increase muscle temperature, metabolic rate, blood flow and lubrication of joints, and to improve muscle contractile capacity. Here are some of the benefits of a good warm-up.

1 Muscle temperature increases, resulting in:
- the muscle contracting more forcefully;
- the muscle relaxing more quickly;
- speed and strength enhancement.

2 The blood temperature increases as blood flows through the warmed-up muscle. This also makes more oxygen available to the muscle.

3 Hormonal changes occur, resulting in:
- a greater production of hormones responsible for regulating energy production;
- more carbohydrate and fatty acids being made available for energy production.

4 The metabolic rate increases, which improves the body's ability to process energy.

The higher the training intensity of a workout, the longer the warm-up should be, for instance 15 to 20 minutes for intervals, 20 to 30 minutes for races. Breaking out in a sweat means that your warm-up is satisfactory, as it indicates that you have raised your body's internal temperature. Stretching should follow the warm-up (see below).

Warm-ups and tiredness

If you have difficulty during the warm-up and workout in reaching your normal steady-state heart rate, or you feel very heavy-legged, this could indicate tiredness; for example, you may experience leg fatigue in your intervals if you are a runner or cyclist. If you can't reach your heart rate in the warm-up you should either go home and rest or continue with a short, active recovery (very low-intensity) workout.

Warm-up stretches

Stretches during warm-up increase your range of movement, thereby allowing you to work out optimally. Stretching can also help prevent injury. Stretches should be specific to the workout. Lack of flexibility can result in inefficient movement, causing loss of speed and poor technique.

Each stretch should be performed in a slow, controlled manner. Move slowly into the stretch until the *first sensation* of a stretch is felt – any more tension in the stretch can cause muscle overstretching, which results in muscle tightening rather than loosening. You should not bounce during the stretch, and no sudden, jerky movements are advised as both can cause injury. Hold each stretch for ten to fifteen seconds (less is not really beneficial) and try to fully relax the muscle being stretched and the surrounding muscles.

Be sensitive to tension in the muscle as this will determine how many repetitions you should perform. This also acts as a guide to improvements in your stretching and prevents overstretching. Be aware of any flexibility imbalances between left and right limbs. Emphasise the less flexible side until balance is achieved. And note that more stretching and a longer warm-up will be required in the morning as you will generally be less flexible at this time of the day.

Warm-down

A warm-down is a drop in exercise intensity designed to promote recovery. It will help prevent blood pooling at your extremities, which can make you feel light-headed (common after speedwork). In a cyclist, for example, blood pools in the blood vessels in the legs and not enough returns to the heart. As a consequence, the heart beats faster in an attempt to increase blood flow. The result? You feel dizzy.

During a workout exercise-induced by-products are accumulated in the body and these affect performance in the following workouts. If you stop exercise cold, by-products remain in the body and removal will take much longer as your metabolic rate (the basic speed at which your body functions) drops to resting. Ideally, you should lower your training intensity to a light activity which does not stress the body, that is, does not produce further by-products. At low training intensities, exercise by-products are removed at a much faster rate as your metabolic rate is still higher than at rest. This will improve the rate of recovery, allowing for 'fresher' and more effective exercise in following workouts. The higher the training intensity used in the workout the longer the warm-down: for example, 20 to 30 minutes for intervals and races.

Warming down after a race can take a lot of discipline – you'd often much rather have a drink, eat and talk – but get that warm-down done first!

Warm-down stretches

This is the best time to develop and improve your flexibility. Warm-down stretching should be targeted at the specific muscles used in the exercise just performed; for example, after a running workout stretch your running muscles. Most flexibility gains are made following exercise. Warm-down stretching is aimed more at improving performance than preventing injury. For example, hamstring (back of thigh) stretches could improve stride length for running which in some cases may improve speed.

For lazy stretchers

Some athletes do not like stretching. If you are one of those athletes, at least try and stretch up to three times per week rather than not at all (it might help to think about which you hate more:

and race distance/intensity. Longer races, such as an Ironman or marathon, may need to be followed by two or three weeks of light activity.

If you have raced for over 20 minutes there should be no speedwork in the week following a race, or at least not until late in the week. Don't forget that a race *is* speedwork. More experienced athletes will recover faster and therefore will be able to start doing their speedwork earlier than less experienced athletes.

If you have muscle soreness following a race, exercise lightly, at a very low intensity, with no muscle stress on the sore muscles. Exercise in a low-impact and fluid form of exercise; for instance, if you have just done a triathlon, don't run with muscle soreness – swim or cycle gently for a short period.

Flexibility and stretching

The accepted reason for stretching is primarily injury prevention through greater flexibility. However, a more important reason for stretching is to improve performance through an increased range of motion and a reduction in fatigue (loose muscles don't fight against each other). Loose muscles contract/relax faster and technique work can be performed more accurately with no limitations due to inflexibility. Flexible muscles also recover more quickly as they suffer less exercise trauma and damage, and have a better blood flow.

Good flexibility is thus an important factor in sports performance. Of course, flexibility varies widely between individuals, but most athletes can benefit from being more flexible than they are. And there's nothing worse than failing to finish an event because of muscle tightness, such as a sore back in rowing, cycling or kayaking.

Muscle imbalances, for example, where the left hamstring is tighter than the right, can also

Missing workouts

In almost every build-up you will miss workouts and training days due to overtiredness or lack of time. This is normal and an expected part of training. An athlete generally misses up to four days/workouts per month, over and above prescribed days off. This varies depending on the individual, but missing workouts is a fact of training life and nothing to get concerned about. If you miss a day unexpectedly, never try to catch up the missed mileage the following day, or do extra on your day off. If a workout is missed, it is gone! It is better to look at a missed day in a positive way – it is both a physical and mental day off. It is a day where your body rests, recovers and improves. Trying to catch up mileage destroys the balance (exercise versus recovery) of the programme and may lead to excessive fatigue and extended negative effects on your training programme.

Listen to your body. If you feel tired, adjust your training to take this into account. Trying to do prescribed mileage in a fatigued state is of no benefit whatsoever. Put another way, resting for a day because of fatigue may mean only one day of training is affected. However, trying to do the workout despite fatigue may affect several days or even weeks of training, with far greater potential for overtraining. Think about it: what would you rather have? One day off or one week off? Now, that's a no-brainer!

If you miss three or four days in a row through tiredness or lack of enthusiasm for training, then it is likely that total mileage or speedwork is too excessive. If not quickly reduced or adjusted, overtraining may occur.

Monitoring your fatigue levels is always the most important guide to training. Listen to your body first, then listen to your coach or follow your programme.

harm performance and may lead to injury if not dealt with.

Either assess your own flexibility while doing your stretching – you may feel tight in a specific area or one limb/side – or get your flexibility checked by a fitness testing lab.

Types of stretching

Static

- Slow, held stretching. The joint is taken to a certain point and held. This form of stretching is particularly recommended.
- PNF (proprioceptive neuromuscular facilitation) stretching is static stretching, but the joint is taken to a point where a mild stretch is felt and then you contract the muscle against the direction of the stretch. The contraction is held for five to ten seconds. The muscle will then be able to be moved through a greater range of motion. This technique is continued until no further movement gains are made for the stretch. PNF is particularly useful for inflexible athletes.

Dynamic

Through forceful movement, the joint/muscle is taken through a greater range of motion than it can normally achieve, for example a high, straight leg kick to stretch the hamstring.

How to stretch

1 Always do a warm-up and warm-down. Don't try and hurry your stretching.
2 You don't have to stretch every muscle every time you stretch (good news if you don't enjoy stretching). Do the stretches that are most specific to the workout. If you need to do a lot of stretches for a particular area, do these in the warm-up and warm-down, with the key area getting the most attention in the warm-down. Split the other stretches between the warm-up and warm-down.
3 Make time to stretch! Many athletes use lack of time as an excuse not to stretch. You're better off cutting your workout by five minutes at each end and stretching than risking injury/poor training performance because you're tight.
4 When stretching, concentrate on technique. Understand where you feel the stretch and aim to reproduce it over and over. As you become more experienced with your stretching you will find that simply assuming a stretching position may not be enough to add to your flexibility. You will then need to look carefully at technique and at fully relaxing the stretched muscle.
5 Move into all stretches slowly and be sensitive to the tension being placed on the stretched muscle. You should slowly move into the stretch until you feel the first sign of comfortable mild tension in the muscle. Hold this for 10 to 15 seconds.
6 Stretching will be enhanced if you are relaxed. Relax not only the muscle groups you are stretching, but your entire body. Stay loose! Stretching is also enhanced if you visualise the muscle being slowly stretched. Imagine you can look inside your leg or arm and see the muscle slowly being stretched out. You may even want to imagine it as a piece of chewing gum or putty. See and feel the muscle slowly and gently being stretched. It's a great feeling!
7 Your muscles are protected by a 'stretch reflex'. This means that if you overstretch a muscle by bouncing or pushing the muscle past its natural elastic capabilities, the muscle's reflex response is to contract (tighten). This contraction stops you from stretching to the point where serious damage could be done.

If you are already very tight in an area, be particularly careful, as overstretching this area will see the muscle contract and get very tight. This may lead to pain and/or injury through microscopic tears in the muscle fibres. These tears can form scar tissue on the muscle and may decrease muscle elasticity. This also occurs if you begin vigorous activity without first warming up. Overstretching actually increases the tightness of the muscle you are trying to loosen!

8 The limb you are stretching should not be shaking due to excessive muscle tension. Don't 'bounce' – controlled movements only.

9 Never try a new stretch before a race! Stick to those you have been doing regularly. A new stretch at this late stage only invites injury or soreness.

10 Be careful stretching during exercise. Generally, your perception of pain drops during exercise so there is a danger you may overstretch without realising you're doing so.

11 Finally, when it comes to stretching, the 'No Pain, No Gain' philosophy *does not apply*. Stretching can improve performance, prevent injury and make your movements more fluid. But only if it is done slowly and gently. A more flexible, supple body is worth working for, but remember that overstretching can be as ineffective as understretching. Bottom line: if you don't relax when you stretch, your flexibility will not improve.

See fig. 6.2 for stretching exercises.

Stretching recommendations

1 rep each side = very flexible
2 reps each side = average flexibility
3 reps each side = below average flexibility
4-6 reps each side = poor flexibility or problem area (e.g. injury)
Note: In the case of flexibility imbalance, more reps should be used on the tighter muscle or limb.

Strength and strength training

Strength is defined as the ability of a muscle group to exert maximal contractile force against a resistance. It is widely regarded as the foundation of speed and endurance. Strength tests on elite endurance athletes appear to indicate that standard gymnasium strength training may not significantly improve performance. Nevertheless, there are many athletes (novice to elite) who will claim that strength training has helped their performance.

Despite this, strength training does appear better suited to short-distance, 'explosive' sports, such as rowing, track riding and sprinting, than to endurance-oriented sports like marathons, tour cycling and Ironman. The best answer is to try strength training for yourself and see if it benefits you. Young athletes should approach strength training with care as it can be harmful, although lighter sport-specific strength training during a workout or use of light weights at high reps is possible.

If you do use strength training, make sure you do it correctly. An important aspect is timing – it should be done early in the buildup, preferably in Base 1 or even in the off-season. This is because strength training will severely fatigue the strength-trained muscles and this in turn will have a major effect on your ability to complete training mileages. In Base 2, as training becomes more sport-specific, strength training is generally discontinued or greatly reduced, for example once or twice a week instead of three or four times, or it may be restricted to a particular body area; a cyclist may continue to work on upper body in Base 2, for example.

As a rule, the shorter and more explosive the race distance, the more strength and bulk

Figure 6.2 Flexibility and stretching exercises

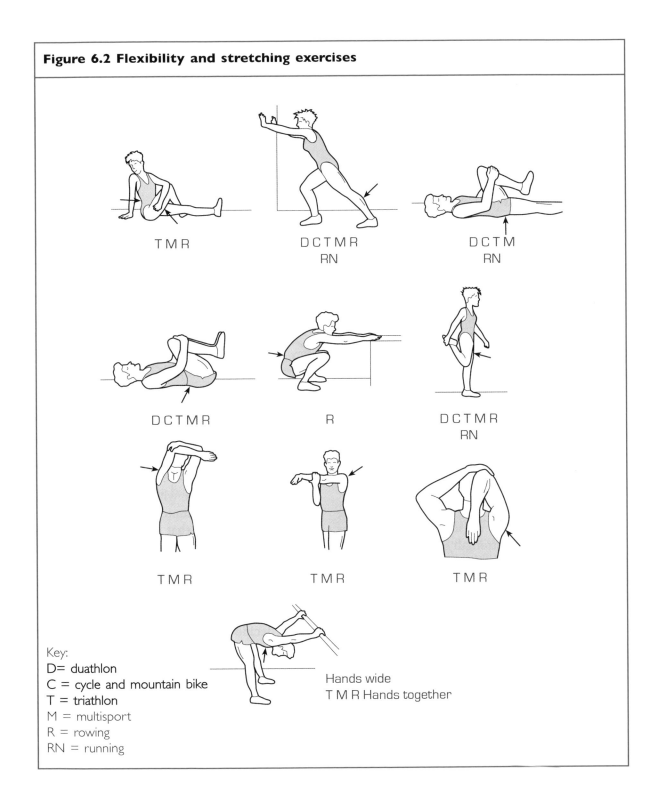

Key:
D= duathlon
C = cycle and mountain bike
T = triathlon
M = multisport
R = rowing
RN = running

Hands wide
T M R Hands together

blood samples and testing for lactic acid concentrations. All of these tests involve a gradual increase in test workload and exercise intensity. Each test will show a marked change when the athlete reaches a predominantly anaerobic state: loss of controlled breathing, heart rate plateaus (causing a deflection on a graph), or a very sudden lactate accumulation (concentration of lactic acid in the blood). Some exercise labs now express AT as a workload, e.g. 200 Watts, as athletes seem to relate well to this measure.

Running test for anaerobic threshold

This running test is a basic way of predicting anaerobic threshold. It is not the most accurate in the world, but it is still a useful guide. This test was developed in 1989 by Dr Art Weltman at the University of Virginia.

The test involves a 3200 m time trial run and can be used to determine the percentage of your maximum you can sustain in a race. It is not specific for non-runners, but can provide a very loose guide to training. Time is measured in minutes, e.g. 30 sec = 0.5 min.

For men: $VO_2 = 122.0 - (5.310 \times \text{time for 3200 m run})$
For women: $VO_2 = (-1.120 \times \text{time for 3200 m run}) + 61.57$ (Note the negative in this equation.)

For example, a 40-year-old male with a 3200 m time of 14 min:

$$
\begin{aligned}
VO_2\text{max} &= 122 - (5.31 \times 14) \\
&= 122 - (74.34) \\
&= 47.66
\end{aligned}
$$

Divide your result (47.66) by your VO_2max (56) and multiply by 100 to reach a percentage figure:

$$(47.66 \div 56) \times 100 = 85\%$$

Therefore, anaerobic threshold is at 85 per cent of VO_2max. See the basic VO_2max test on page 112 for information on calculating your VO_2max.

Conconi test

This test is very strenuous, so get medical clearance if you are unsure about your ability to cope with it, particularly if you are over the age of 35.

One of the more notable experts in developing techniques for testing anaerobic threshold was an Italian physician and physiologist named Francesco Conconi. He developed a method for determining anaerobic threshold without needing to take blood samples. This was achieved by monitoring the athlete's heart rate as he or she steadily increased exercise effort. Conconi and his test became very famous when it was used successfully to train a cyclist named Francesco Moser to break the World One-Hour Cycling record.

The advantage of the Conconi test is that it is very simple, does not require a lot of expensive testing equipment and, with the help of a couple of assistants, you can conduct it yourself.

Runners (including run discipline in triathlon)

You will need:

- an accurate heart rate monitor;
- two helpers, one equipped with a stopwatch and the other with a bike set up with a bike computer that measures kph – the bike can be optional;
- a 200 m indoor track (or 400 m outdoor track but test in windless conditions).

Measure and mark a section of track 50 m in length (for 400 m track mark two 50 m sections 200 m apart).

After a good warm-up (at least 20 min) start the test running with the cyclist at a very comfortable pace. Run behind or beside the bike around the track (preferably beside bike on outside). The cyclist must maintain an even speed throughout each lap. The cyclist is there to control the runner's pace and speed exactly, using a cycle computer. After each 200 m lap the cyclist must increase the pace for the runner by 0.5 kph (if testing without a cyclist, increase running speed by 5 seconds per kilometre).

The second helper will be timing the final 50 m of each 200 m section so your actual running speed can be determined and to double check the cycle computer. Each time you pass the end of the marked 50 m call out your heart rate. Your assistant will record the heart rate next to the time for that 50 m section (there are monitors available that will record this so you don't have call out heart rates). Continue until you feel that you have passed your anaerobic threshold (once heart rate is no longer increasing as fast as running speed, breathing frequency dramatically increases and you find it difficult or impossible to increase your pace further).

Cyclists/mountain bikers (including cycle discipline in triathlon)

You will need:

- accurate heart rate monitor;
- an assistant to record heart rates/speeds;
- a bike computer that measures speed and cadence;
- a velodrome (choose a windless day) or a stationary cycle trainer.

Warm up for 10 to 20 minutes. Each lap should be between 300 and 450 m. If you use a windtrainer, use an appropriate time interval (30–50 sec between speed increases). You can change gears if you are an experienced cyclist (cadence must remain constant though); if you are not experienced you should start in a moderately large gear and not gear change during the test. Ride in your racing position and maintain constant pace during each lap. Increase your speed by 1 or 2 kph for each lap (use the same increase each lap.) Keep increasing the speed until your legs are too tired to continue. At the end of each lap call out your heart rate so that it can be recorded by your assistant.

Note: triathletes need to test both running and cycling anaerobic threshold as the heart rates and speeds recorded may be vastly different. Tests should be conducted on separate days with enough time to recover fully in between. These protocols can be adapted for kayaking, swimming and rowing but practicalities make tests more difficult to conduct.

Calculate your speed (running or cycling) per section of lap (refer to 'Useful Calculations', appendix 1). On a graph, plot your recorded heart rates on the vertical axis and your speed on the horizontal axis. If your test has gone as planned, your graph should show an evenly sloping line until the point where your heart rate was unable to increase at the same rate as speed – your heart rate plateau (*see* fig. 6.3). These zones on the graph just before and just after where the sloping line deflects are the top and bottom heart rates for your anaerobic threshold zone (preferably a five to ten beat range). You can record your test results and plot them on a graph.

Test every two to eight weeks towards the end of an easy week in your mesocycles. Rest for 18 to 24 hours before the test to freshen up. Test every two weeks in the speed phase and every eight weeks in the base phase. Figure 6.4 shows how your anaerobic threshold can change.

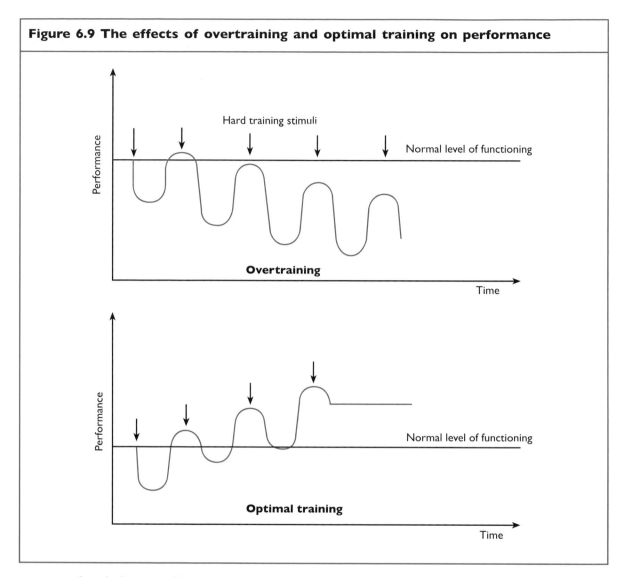

Figure 6.9 The effects of overtraining and optimal training on performance

too soon, break down and lose interest, or they are unable to train at the levels they once did because of continuing health problems.

Adaptation via a slow controlled increase in training volume and intensity is the aim of any good training programme. If given the chance, the body has an amazing ability to adapt and improve its performance through training.

While overtraining is a common problem in endurance athletes, particularly athletes training for ultra-distance races and those who race often, it also occurs in athletes who try to fit training in around work and social obligations and leave little time for recovery (physical and mental). Overtraining can occur through heavy training mileages towards the end of base training, during intensive speed training or after a series of races within a short period of time.

Causes of overtraining

Overtraining needs to be differentiated from the short-term tiredness that occurs whenever training load increases. Overtrained athletes may be doing no more training than their peers, but due to outside pressures, medical problems or even their personal tolerance to training, may be feeling fatigued. Remember, to achieve performance improvement, the body must be allowed to adapt gradually to increased training mileages and intensities. But it is not absolute mileages and intensities that matter, but rather the amount of mileage and speedwork you personally can recover from – no recovery, no improvement!

Causes of overtraining

Main causes

1. Inadequate recovery between training sessions
2. Excessive amounts of high-intensity (and sometimes high-volume) training
3. Sudden changes in training load (distance, duration or intensity)

Other training factors that contribute to overtraining

1. Intense strength training
2. Frequent competition and travel
3. Monotony in training programme
4. No off-season

Non-training factors that contribute to overtraining

1. Inadequate nutrition
2. Insufficient sleep and rest
3. Anxiety about life events, e.g. new job
4. Occupational stress
5. Mental conflict
6. Changes and irregularities in lifestyle
7. Successive failure to achieve goals

Your ability to recover, of course, depends largely on your training history. The more years you have been in the sport, the bigger your base, the more training you can do and recover from. Elite athletes are particularly susceptible to overtraining as double seasons (winter and summer) can mean an inadequate off-season with too little time for recovery. Young athletes and inexperienced athletes are also susceptible to overtraining because of their lower tolerance to training. Common training errors that lead to overtraining are too long a season, high levels of competitive stress, frequent racing, intense training over an extended period of time, lack of effective recovery and lack of positive results/enjoyment.

Symptoms of overtraining

Emotional and behavioural changes

- Lethargy and excessive fatigue, especially at rest
- Loss of purpose, energy and competitive drive; poor attitude, confusion, loss of enthusiasm to train
- Feelings of helplessness and being trapped in routine
- Feeling emotionally unstable and excessive emotional display
- Loss of libido (loss of interest in sex)
- Increased anxiety and depressive feelings
- Increased irritability and anger (mood changes)
- Sleep problems (difficulty getting to sleep, nightmares, waking often during the night)
- Decreased self-confidence
- Poor concentration, inability to relax

Physical changes

- Weight loss, weight fluctuations and loss of appetite
- Heavy painful muscles, 'weak-feeling' muscles
- Excessive sweating

PART **TWO**

TAKING IT TO THE NEXT LEVEL

HOW TO WRITE YOUR OWN PROGRAMME

7

Set realistic training goals

Goal setting improves motivation, but only if the goal is realistic and achievable. When planning your training programme, set yourself realistic intermediate and long-term goals in terms of how much and how fast. It is always tempting to set training goals that you would *like* to achieve rather than those you *can* achieve at this point in your sporting career. Unattainable goals may look good on paper, but they can lead to overtraining and decrease motivation as you fail to achieve them. Of course, if you have already been training for several seasons and have been keeping a training log, then you should have a good idea of what you can handle when it comes to races, training volume and training intensity. Use this hard-earned knowledge to establish effective training seasons and periods.

For most athletes, increases in training volume should not exceed 10 or, at the most, 15 per cent over a season. Remember, there is a limit to how much training you can do no matter how much time and motivation you have at your disposal! So, set goals you can achieve, be patient and don't become a slave to your programme. If in doubt, back off and regroup. You'll be a happier, healthier athlete for doing so. I don't advise setting training programmes of more than 14 weeks. The busier you are, the shorter the programme should be.

The three levels of your training programme

When planning a training programme three levels are used. These are:

1 Blueprint – the plan, what you would like to do
2 Working programme – what you actually do; 'the real world'
3 Log book – what happened.

1 Blueprint

The blueprint outlines your overall training plan for the year (or longer), including specific details about build-up and racing. This blueprint is your ideal plan and as such will prove almost impossible to follow to the letter. Fatigue, illness, lack of time, work, family, study and so on can, and will probably, all have an adverse effect on training type, intensity and duration at some stage during the year. Don't worry. The blueprint is only a guide as to how to approach your training programme and achieve training goals. It is not your definitive training programme.

2 Working programme

A working programme is the weekly programme recorded at the end of each week. It takes into account:

- Blueprint
- Next week's commitments

- You and/or your coach's requirements for the week
- Your experience
- Information from the log book and any other relevant information from the previous week's training

Combined, these elements are used to determine each week's programme (*see* fig. 7.1). It's called the working programme because it's the programme that actually 'works'. It almost certainly won't follow the blueprint exactly and will include subtle changes and refinements from week to week as circumstances change and your experience grows. For a step-by-step guide on how to complete your working programme *see* page 164.

3 The log book

The log book is a combination of the previous year's blueprint, past weekly training programmes, monthly summaries and post-peak analysis summaries (summary of complete build-up).

The log book is used to see exactly what happened in previous build-ups, what effect the training had on performance, and to identify long-term trends in training. The log book, therefore, is used to develop the next blueprint, including the week-to-week programme.

How to set up your blueprint

Training programmes must be set up in a logical order. This involves setting up the blueprint first.

Step 1: Set up your 'seasonal programme'

Your seasonal programme includes: off-season, pre-season, in-season. To set up the programme you will need to decide the exact dates of the races you wish to compete in, and the length of those races (longer races require longer build-ups, meaning fewer races can be raced in a season). Once you have these dates, set out your seasonal programme following the example

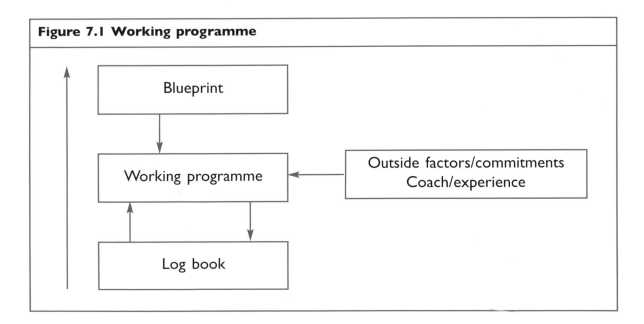

Figure 7.1 Working programme

Blueprint

Working programme ← Outside factors/commitments Coach/experience

Log book

given in figure 7.2. To work out how long your seasons should be refer to the relevant sections earlier in the book.

Step 2: Set up your microcycle

Now you need to set up your microcycle (the format for a standard training week), i.e. what training you do on each day. To do this you first need to work out your 'peak-mileage week'.

Your peak-mileage week

Your peak-mileage (or duration) week is the week in your build-up in which you do the greatest volume (hours or kilometres) of training. This is *not* a weekly average. It is the mileage for one week only. You may only do this week once or twice in your entire build-up (near the end of base, or early in speedwork),

as it is the culmination of a gradual build-up of volume over a long time.

To work this out, simply calculate the biggest weekly mileage you think you could cope with, given your experience, commitment, time and ability to avoid injury, in all the disciplines you intend to compete in. For example, let's imagine you are an elite runner with ten years' experience of high training loads. You might decide that your peak-mileage week will be 160 km. Alternatively, you might be a novice triathlete in your second season of competing, who also works full-time. You might decide that you can only cope with a maximum of six hours' training per week spread across swimming, cycling and running. If training for a multi-disciplinary sport, such as triathlon, generally you are better off to establish training mileages or durations for each discipline.

You can determine your own 'peak-mileage

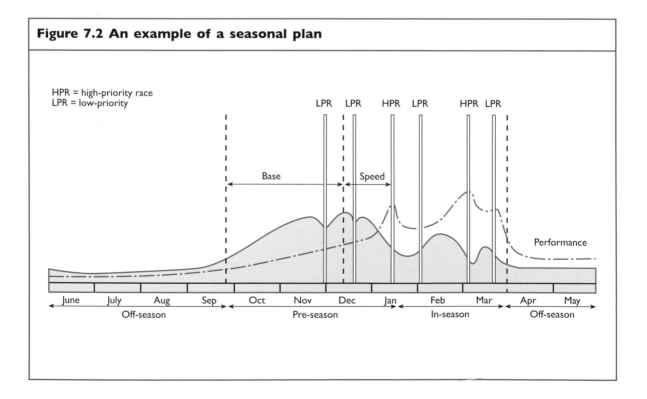

Figure 7.2 An example of a seasonal plan

HPR = high-priority race
LPR = low-priority

Figure 7.3 Example of a peak mileage week

Standard weekly training format

Sport	Mon	Tue	Wed	Thurs	Fri	Sat	Sun	Total
Swim	2 km		2 km		Day Off	1.5 km		5.5 km
Bike		40 km (speed)		40 km (hills)	Day Off		80 km (long)	160 km
Run	16 km (hills)		20 km (long)		Day Off	10 km (speed)		46 km

week', or if you need help Section A (*see* pages 143–145) provides guidelines to work out your peak-mileage week based on your sport, the distance you intend to race, and your level of training commitment. Whatever you decide, remember it is best to be cautious. Fill in your peak-mileage week total (or totals if you plan to compete in more than one discipline) following the example in figure 7.3.

Now you have to decide how to spread that

Figure 7.4 Weekly build-up programme template

Standard weekly training format

Week	1	2	3	4	5	6	7	8	9	10	11	12	13	14
Date														
Mesocycle														
%														
Sport 1														
Sport 2														
Sport 3														

Set up your week-to-week training mileages and periodisation (base/speed/taper) using this table. Work backwards from your goal race, and include lower priority races that you will use as training races.

peak mileage (or duration) throughout the week. In other words, what training you will do on each day. When making your decision take account of work, study, family and social factors, as well as availability of resources, such as pool times, daylight for cycling, training partners and so on. Also take account of the need for a rest day or a day that is very easy. For many people, Friday fits the bill nicely as it comes at the end of the working week and provides a chance to socialise and regroup before the weekend, when much of your mileage work is likely to be done.

Table 7.1 provides an example of how a triathlete might spread 211.5 km (swim 5.5 km, bike 160 km, run 46 km) of training across a week.

If you are an experienced athlete, you will probably have a good idea as to how to set up your microcycle for a peak-mileage week. When setting up a microcycle, work it out in the following order:

1 Day or days off
2 Workout days
3 Long or medium long workouts
4 Speed workouts
5 Hill workouts
6 Other easy workouts

If you need help, there are pre-set peak-mileage week microcycles for a range of sports and distances in Section B (*see* pages 146–156).

The peak-mileage weeks in Section A have numbers next to them which correspond to the training weeks in Section B. If using Section B, remember to select a pre-set programme based on your sport, the distance you intend racing over and the level of training that suits you. These programmes are set up in terms of daily workouts, experience levels, number of workouts per week and mileage for each workout during your *peak-mileage week* only. The programmes can be converted to duration rather than mileage by using Section D (*see* page 162). The times are only approximate, however, and you will need to adjust them according to your ability and experience.

As your peak-mileage week represents the most training you think you can handle in one week, it equates to your 100 per cent week. All other training weeks are based on this week. If you are not experienced in your sport, make sure you select a programme that is realistic in terms of your training experience and non-training commitments. If you have limited time available, you may want to choose a programme based simply on the number of workouts per week. Select a programme based on what you think you can do, not based on what you would like to be doing or what your friends/clubmates are doing. Dreams are free but overtraining is costly. Select wisely!

Table 7.1	Microcycle morning and afternoon adjustments						
Mon	Tues	Wed	Thurs	Fri	Sat	Sun
S 2 km		S 2 km		D/O	S 1.5 km	
	B 40 km		B 40 km	D/O		B 80 km
R 16 km		R 20 km		D/O	R 10 km	

Key: S = swim; B = bike; R = run

Levels of training commitment

You need to select your level from the categories below before choosing peak-mileage and training weeks from Sections A and B.

1 **Recreational/novice**
   - You want to get the most out of little training time because you can't commit to too much training.
   - You are in your first year of the sport.

2 **Semi-competitive**
   - You are prepared to invest a moderate level of commitment. You are serious about training but you have other commitments and interests. You are interested in becoming competitive but you aren't aiming at coming first.
   - You are in your second year of competing and happy to remain at this level of commitment.
   - Having fun is more important than doing 'really well'.

3 **Elite**
   - You are either a top young athlete, a talented athlete new to the sport, or a top athlete who works 40 hours per week. You are serious about your sport and want to place well.
   - You have been competing for three or more years and you are placing well (top 10 or better in most races).

4 **Elite-plus**
   - You are a very serious athlete who trains full-time in order to win!
   - You have been competing for over four years and have already won big races.

Once you have chosen the programme from Section B that you think suits you best, complete a peak mileage week table by filling in each day's training mileage/duration for each of the disciplines you plan to compete in. Figure 7.3 illustrates a peak-mileage week based on the template. You may need to juggle the days around your personal and work schedule. In figure 7.3, for instance, you might not be able to do a long run on Wednesday because of a weekly meeting. Swap it with one of the other running days, but make sure it doesn't upset the balance of the programme. Remember, this is only your peak-mileage week and the basis for working out all other weeks.

You have now filled out your seasonal plan (including race dates), your peak-mileage week total and how much mileage (duration) you are going to do on each day of this week.

Your weekly and daily workouts

You now need to fill in the template in fig. 7.4 or 7.5. On these templates, you will need to count back from your 'Full Peak' race day and fill in the date for Monday of each week during your training build-up.

You now need to work out how much mileage you do each week in your race build-up based on a percentage of your peak-mileage (100 per cent) week. For example, if week two is a 50 per cent week, that means all your workouts in week two are 50 per cent of the distance/duration of those workouts in your peak-mileage week. To find these percentages use Section C (*see* pages 157–161). Even if you have set up the rest of your programme by yourself, it's worth looking at Section C to get an idea of how you can use it. You will see that it provides training percentages based on:

1 Number of weeks of speedwork (four, six or eight)
2 Mesocycle (hard/easy week ratio: 2:1; 3:1; 4:1)
3 Percentage of training volume increase (7 per cent or 10 per cent)
4 Race distance (short or long).

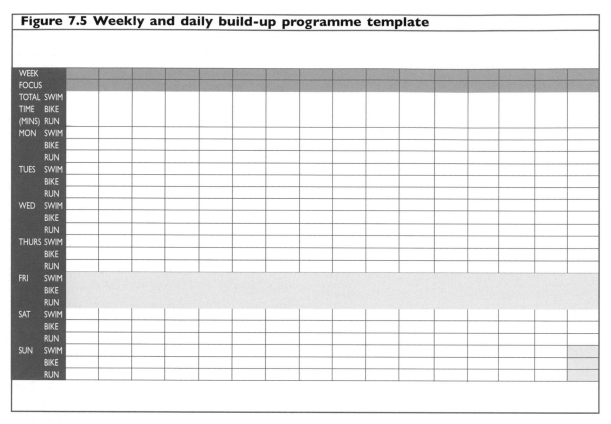

Figure 7.5 Weekly and daily build-up programme template

You now need to select an option for each of these variables. To help you make your selection, consider the following:

1 Number of weeks of speedwork
Four weeks is recommended for beginners and eight weeks for experienced elite athletes. Most athletes will lie in the four- to six-week range. Section C offers three blocks (A, B, C). Block A = four weeks of speedwork; block B = six weeks of speedwork; block C = eight weeks of speedwork. Select the number of weeks that you feel suits you best.

2 Mesocycle (hard/easy weeks)
Remember, a mesocycle is the number of hard weeks (high volumes of distance/duration in base, high volumes of intensity in speed) in a row you can cope with before a recovery or compensation week. A ratio of two hard/one easy is recommended for beginners and four hard/one easy for elite athletes. Choose the option you feel comfortable with (if in doubt, be conservative). You will see that each block offers a mesocycle option. Choose the mesocycle from the block you selected in (1) above.

Ideally, although this option isn't shown in these basic tables, mesocycles change during a build-up, going from smaller cycles (two hard/one easy) to larger cycles (four hard/one easy) in base as you become better conditioned. Then as you move into speedwork the cycle gets smaller again to accommodate the increasing training intensity. You need to be particularly careful at this time that your programme allows you sufficient recovery.

3 Percentage increase per week

If you are experienced, 10 per cent is acceptable, but if you are less experienced, then 7 per cent is the best option. Ideally, and again this option isn't shown in these tables, your programme will start off with smaller increases (as you get used to training), with larger increases in the middle, and then smaller increases again at the end (you can't keep increasing mileage indefinitely!). Select the percentage option from the block you chose earlier (A, B, or C).

4 Race distance

A race is long if it is over three-and-a-half hours, short if it is under. Choose short or long from the block you have chosen.

Here's an example using Section C of how these choices determine your daily training distances or durations:

1 Number of weeks of speedwork = 6
  Go to Block B
2 Mesocycle = 2 hard/1 easy
  Go to lines A–D
3 Percentage increase per week = 10 per cent
  Go to line C or D
4 Race distance = short
  Go to line D.

Line D gives you the percentages you will use to calculate your weekly training distances through build-up and speedwork.

You will notice the programme allows for a base of up to 18 weeks (plus the six weeks of speedwork chosen in this example). You will also notice that some of the weeks indicate your 100 per cent or peak-mileage week, upon which all other weekly mileages are based.

You can start anywhere in the programme.

If you do not wish to do a structured eighteen-week build-up, or are unable to, then start your build-up in later weeks, e.g. start in week seven. Just make sure you give yourself enough time to prepare adequately for the speedwork to come.

If you are not starting a programme at the beginning, make sure your first week of the programme corresponds to current training volumes. You can't just jump into the middle of a programme unfit and expect it to work! The best approach is to determine the number of weeks until you race and then count back until you reach the week you are currently in. If the mileages in the programme equate to what you are doing now, start there. If they are greater than you are doing now, you may need to make some programme adjustments (*see* page 140).

Okay, so you've made your personal choices concerning speedwork, mesocycle and percentage increase. Now go back to the template in fig. 7.4 and fill in the percentage line. Note that in most instances the lines in the percentage ranges at the end of build-up – weeks 23 or 24 – in Section C are excluded, as you should use the taper programmes presented in Part 3.

Now complete the template for each week, and each discipline by multiplying your peak-mileage week total by the percentage you wrote for each week, e.g. bike 160 km x 72 (0.72) = 115 km. This gives you the mileage you will do each week for each discipline. Write these totals on the appropriate lines. For example, if the percentage in week 1 is 72 per cent you will see that this means in base week 1 you would do: 4 km swimming, 115 km cycling, 33 km running. Note: 72 per cent would not be an appropriate starting point for a novice; 40 per cent would be more appropriate.

Once you have got mileages (or durations)

3 Approximate 'in-season' adjustments. In-season involves manipulation of base and speed training. Ideally, your peak races need to be six to eight weeks apart to enable you to peak effectively (100 per cent potential). In such cases, the approximate plan would be two to four weeks of base immediately after the race, including a recovery week, with a little speedwork after the recovery week. The build-up to moderate to high mileage is gradual. Following this, three to five weeks of full speed-work should be implemented to make up the six to eight weeks. A longer race would best suit five weeks of base and three weeks of speed (because of the race distance), while a short race would involve three weeks of base and five weeks of speed (because speed is more important in a shorter race).

For adjustments to training if you have less than six weeks between races, see 'How to manage training during the 'in-season'' on page 70. Remember to use the sport-specific programmes outlined previously so you can work out your requirements for speedwork, long workouts, hills etc., and appropriate tapers.

The basic programme is now in place. Remember that the blueprint is a guide only; it is designed to provide you with a framework to build your training around. And it is this training that gives you the working programme, which we look at in the next chapter.

Table 7.2(a)	Programme adjustment example 1						
Week	1	2	3	4	5	6	7	8
Scheduled %	60	65	70	60	75	80	85	90
Adjusted %	40	50	60	40	65	75	85	90

Table 7.2(b)	Programme adjustment example 2						
Week	1	2	3	4	5	6	7	8
Scheduled %	40	50	60	40	65	75	85	90
Adjusted %	40	50	60	40	65	60	70	90

Section A: Peak-mileage weeks

Use the tables in this section as a guide to work out your peak-mileage week. Note: 2x, 3x, 4x etc. are the number of times you train in each discipline each week; S = swim, B = bike, R = run, K = kayak, Ro = row.

Triathlon

Table 7.3(a)	Peak mileage week for sprint-distance triathlon (700 m/20 km/6 km)			
		S (km)	B (km)	R (km)
Novice	2x	3	70	16
Semi	3x	5.5	120	22
Elite	4x	10	180	34

Table 7.3(b)	Peak mileage week for standard-distance triathlon (1.5 km/40 km/10 km)			
		S (km)	B (km)	R (km)
Novice	2x	3	100	25
Semi	3x	5.5	160	46
Elite	4x	10.5	280	49
Elite+	5x	12.5	310	55

Table 7.3(c)	Peak mileage week for Half Ironman triathlon (2 km/90 km/21 km)			
		S (km)	B (km)	R (km)
Semi	3x	8	220	62
Elite	4x	11	320	69
Elite+	5x	13	350	75

Table 7.3(d)	Peak mileage week for Ironman triathlon (3.8 km/180 km/42 km)			
		S (km)	B (km)	R (km)
Semi	3x	9	280	66
Elite	4x	11	380	79
Elite+	5x	13	410	89

Duathlon

Table 7.4(a)	Peak mileage week for duathlon (4 km/20 km/4 km)		
		B (km)	R (km)
Novice	3x	90	24
Semi	4x	160	38
Elite	5x	250	45

Table 7.4(b)	Peak mileage week for duathlon (10 km/ 60 km/10 km)		
		B (km)	R (km)
Novice	3x	170	42
Semi	4x	260	63
Elite	5x	250	45

Cycling and mountain biking

Table 7.5(a)	Peak mileage week for 40 km cycle/ mountain bike race	
		B (km)
Novice	3x	160
Semi	4x	220
Semi	5x	260
Semi	6x	350
Elite	6x	400

Table 7.5(b)	Peak mileage week for 40 km cycle/ mountain bike race	
		B (km)
Novice	4x	240
Semi	5x	280
Semi	6x	390
Elite	6x	470

Table 7.5(c)	Peak mileage week for 160 km cycle/ mountain bike race	
		B (km)
Novice	4x	280
Semi	5x	380
Semi	6x	450
Elite	6x	560
Elite+	6x	700

Table 7.5(d)	Peak mileage week for cycle/mountain bike tour	
		B (km)
Semi		560
Elite		680
Elite+		850

Rowing

Table 7.6	Peak mileage week for rowing (coxed 4, 2000 m)	
		Ro (km)
Novice	5x	42
Semi	6x	57
Elite	6x	100

Distance running

Table 7.7(a)	Peak mileage week for 10 km	
		R (km)
Novice	3x	32
Novice	4x	42
Semi	5x	58
Semi	6x	64
Elite	6x	87

Table 7.7(b)	Peak mileage week for half-marathon	
		R (km)
Novice	4x	53
Semi	5x	70
Semi	6x	84
Elite	6x	92

Table 7.7(c)	Peak mileage week for marathon	
		R (km)
Novice	4x	66
Semi	5x	88
Semi	6x	94
Elite	6x	113

Section B: Peak-mileage week microcycles

Use this section as a guide to work out how you will spread your training during your 'Peak-mileage week' (100%). The daily workouts for each discipline are listed, top to bottom, in the order they should be done; in the case of duathlon training programmes this may involve a run/bike/run format. When referring to the elite programmes in Section B, the underlined workouts are kept if you are doing the elite+ programme, and eliminated if you are doing the elite programme.

Triathlon

Sprint-distance triathlon (700 m/20 km/5 km)

Table 7.8(a)	Microcycle morning and afternoon adjustments					
Mon	Tues	Wed	Thurs	Fri	Sat	Sun
S 2 km	D/O			D/O	S 1 km	
	D/O	B 10 km		D/O		B 60 km
	D/O		R 10 km	D/O	R 6 km	

Table 7.8(b)	Peak mileage week microcycle for sprint-distance triathlon (700 m/20 km/5 km): semi-competitive 3x					
Mon	Tues	Wed	Thurs	Fri	Sat	Sun
S 2 km		S 2 km		D/O	S 1.5 km	
	B 30 km		B 30 km	D/O		B 60 km
R 6 km	R 10 km		D/O	R 6 km		

Table 7.8(c)	Peak mileage week microcycle for sprint-distance triathlon (700 m/20 km/5 km): elite 4x					
Mon	Tues	Wed	Thurs	Fri	Sat	Sun
S 3 km		S 3 km		S 3 km	S 1 km	
	B 40 km		B 40 km		B 20 km	B 80 km
R 10 km		R 15 km			R 6 km	R 3 km

Standard-distance triathlon (1.5 km/40 km/10 km)

| Table 7.9(a) | Peak mileage week microcycle for standard-distance triathlon (1.5 km/40 km/10 km): novice 2x | | | | | |
Mon	Tues	Wed	Thurs	Fri	Sat	Sun
S 1.5 km	D/O			D/O	S 1.5 km	
	D/O	B 40 km		D/O		B 60 km
	D/O		R 15 km	D/O	R 10 km	

| Table 7.9(b) | Peak mileage week microcycle for standard-distance triathlon (1.5 km/40 km/10 km): semi-competitive 3x | | | | | |
Mon	Tues	Wed	Thurs	Fri	Sat	Sun
S 2 km		S 2 km		D/O	S 1.5 km	
	B 40 km		B 40 km	D/O		B 80 km
R 16 km		R 20 km		D/O	R 10 km	

| Table 7.9(c) | Peak mileage week microcycle for standard-distance triathlon (1.5 km/40 km/10 km): elite 4x/elite+ 5x | | | | | |
Mon	Tues	Wed	Thurs	Fri	Sat	Sun
S 3 km	S 2 km	S 3 km		S 3 km	S 1.5 km	
	B 60 km	B 30 km	B 60 km		B 40 km	B 120 km
R 16 km		R 20 km	R 6 km		R 10 km	R 3 km

Half Ironman (2 km/90 km/21 km)

Table 7.10(a)	Peak mileage week microcycle for Half-Ironman (2 km/90 km/21 km): semi-competitive 3					
Mon	Tues	Wed	Thurs	Fri	Sat	Sun
S 3 km		S 3 km		D/O	S 2 km	
	B 60 km		B 60 km	D/O		B 100 km
R 16 km		R 26 km		D/O	R 20 km	

Table 7.10(b)	Peak mileage week microcycle for Half-Ironman (2 km/90 km/21 km): elite 4x/elite+ 5x					
Mon	Tues	Wed	Thurs	Fri	Sat	Sun
S 3 km	S 2 km	S 3 km		S 3 km	S 2 km	
	B 60 km	B 30 km	B 80 km		B 40 km	B 140 km
R 16 km		R 30 km	R 6 km		R 20 km	R 3 km

Ironman (3.8 km/180 km/42 km)

Table 7.11(a)	Peak mileage week microcycle for Ironman (3.8 km/180 km/42 km): semi-competitive 3x					
Mon	Tues	Wed	Thurs	Fri	Sat	Sun
S 3 km		S 3 km		D/O	S 3 km	
	B 40 km		B 60 km	D/O		B 180 km
R 20 km		R 30 km		D/O	R 16 km	

Table 7.11(b)	Peak mileage week microcycle for Ironman (3.8 km/180 km/42 km): elite 4x/elite+ 5x					
Mon	Tues	Wed	Thurs	Fri	Sat	Sun
S 3 km	S 2 km	S 3 km		S 3 km	S 2 km	
	B 80 km	B 30 km	B 60 km		B 60 km	B 180 km
R 20 km		R 36 km	R 10 km		R 20 km	R 3 km

Duathlon

4 km/20 km/4 km duathlon

Table 7.12(a)	Peak mileage week microcycle for duathlon (4 km/20 km/4 km): novice 3x					
Mon	Tues	Wed	Thurs	Fri	Sat	Sun
D/O	R 6 km		R 10 km	D/O	R 4 km	
D/O		B 30 km		D/O	B 20 km	B 40 km
D/O				D/O	R 4 km	

Table 7.12(b)	Peak mileage week microcycle for duathlon (4 km/20 km/4 km): semi-competitive 4x					
Mon	Tues	Wed	Thurs	Fri	Sat	Sun
R 10 km		R 18 km		D/O	R 4 km	R 2 km
	B 40 km		B 40 km	D/O	B 20 km	B 60 km
				D/O	R 4 km	

Table 7.12(c)	Peak mileage week microcycle for duathlon (4 km/20 km/4 km): elite to elite+ 5x					
Mon	Tues	Wed	Thurs	Fri	Sat	Sun
R 10 km		R 18 km	R 6 km	D/O	R 4 km	R 3 km
	B 40 km	B 30 km	B 60 km	D/O	B 20 km	B 100 km
				D/O	R 4 km	

10 km/60 km/10 km duathlon

Table 7.13(a)	Peak mileage week microcycle for duathlon (10 km/60 km/10 km): novice 3x					
Mon	Tues	Wed	Thurs	Fri	Sat	Sun
D/O	R 20 km		R 10 km	D/O	R 6 km	
D/O		B 40 km		D/O	B 30 km	B 100 km
D/O				D/O	R 6 km	

160 km cycle

Table 7.16(a)	Peak mileage week microcycle for cycling (160 km): novice 4x					
Mon	Tues	Wed	Thurs	Fri	Sat	Sun
D/O	40 km	D/O	60 km	D/O	40 km	140 km

Table 7.16(b)	Peak mileage week microcycle for cycling (160 km): semi-competitive 5x					
Mon	Tues	Wed	Thurs	Fri	Sat	Sun
D/O	60 km	40 km	80 km	D/O	40 km	160 km

Table 7.16(c)	Peak mileage week microcycle for cycling (160 km): semi-competitive 6x					
Mon	Tues	Wed	Thurs	Fri	Sat	Sun
30 km	80 km	40 km	80 km	D/O	60 km	160 km

Table 7.16(d)	Peak mileage week microcycle for cycling (160 km): elite 6x					
Mon	Tues	Wed	Thurs	Fri	Sat	Sun
40 km	100 km	60 km	80 km	D/O	80 km	200 km

Table 7.16(e)	Peak mileage week microcycle for cycling (160 km): elite+ 6x					
Mon	Tues	Wed	Thurs	Fri	Sat	Sun
80 km	160 km	40 km	130 km	D/O	90 km	200 km

Cycling tour

Table 7.17(a)	Peak mileage week microcycle for cycling (tour): semi-competitive 6x						
Mon	Tues	Wed	Thurs	Fri	Sat	Sun
40 km	100 km	60 km	100 km	D/O	80 km	180 km

Table 7.17(b)	Peak mileage week microcycle for cycling (tour): elite 6x						
Mon	Tues	Wed	Thurs	Fri	Sat	Sun
60 km	160 km	40 km	130 km	D/O	90 km	200 km

Table 7.17(c)	Peak mileage week microcycle for cycling (tour): elite+ 6x						
Mon	Tues	Wed	Thurs	Fri	Sat	Sun
80 km	160 km	130 km	160 km	D/O	120 km	200 km

Rowing

Table 7.18(a)	Peak mileage week microcycle for rowing (coxed 4, 2000 m): novice 5x						
Mon	Tues	Wed	Thurs	Fri	Sat	Sun
D/O	6 km	10 km	6 km	D/O	10 km	10 km

Table 7.18(b)	Peak mileage week microcycle for rowing (coxed 4, 2000 m): semi-competitive 6x						
Mon	Tues	Wed	Thurs	Fri	Sat	Sun
6 km	10 km	6 km	10 km	D/O	10 km	15 km

Table 7.18(c)	Peak mileage week microcycle for rowing (coxed 4, 2000 m): elite to elite+ 6x						
Mon	Tues	Wed	Thurs	Fri	Sat	Sun
12 km	17 km	12 km	17 km	D/O	23 km	19 km

153

Distance running
10 km run

Table 7.19(a)	Peak mileage week microcycle for 10 km run: novice 3x					
Mon	Tues	Wed	Thurs	Fri	Sat	Sun
D/O	6 km	D/O	10 km	D/O	D/O	16 km

Table 7.19(b)	Peak mileage week microcycle for 10 km run: novice 4x					
Mon	Tues	Wed	Thurs	Fri	Sat	Sun
D/O	10 km	D/O	10 km	D/O	6 km	16 km

Table 7.19(c)	Peak mileage week microcycle for 10 km run: semi-competitive 5x					
Mon	Tues	Wed	Thurs	Fri	Sat	Sun
D/O	16 km	6 km	10 km	D/O	6 km	20 km

Table 7.19(d)	Peak mileage week microcycle for 10 km run: semi-competitive 6x					
Mon	Tues	Wed	Thurs	Fri	Sat	Sun
6 km	16 km	6 km	10 km	D/O	6 km	20 km

Table 7.19(e)	Peak mileage week microcycle for 10 km run: elite to elite+ 6x					
Mon	Tues	Wed	Thurs	Fri	Sat	Sun
6 km	18 km	10 km	16 km	D/O	12 km	25 km

Half-marathon

Table 7.20(a)	Peak mileage week microcycle for half-marathon: novice 4x					
Mon	Tues	Wed	Thurs	Fri	Sat	Sun
D/O	10 km	D/O	16 km	D/O	6 km	21 km

Table 7.20(b)	Peak mileage week microcycle for half-marathon: semi-competitive 5x					
Mon	Tues	Wed	Thurs	Fri	Sat	Sun
D/O	14 km	6 km	18 km	D/O	6 km	26 km

Table 7.20(c)	Peak mileage week microcycle for half-marathon: semi-competitive 6x					
Mon	Tues	Wed	Thurs	Fri	Sat	Sun
6 km	16 km	10 km	20 km	D/O	6 km	26 km

Table 7.20(d)	Peak mileage week microcycle for half-marathon: elite to elite+ 6x					
Mon	Tues	Wed	Thurs	Fri	Sat	Sun
8 km	16 km	10 km	20 km	D/O	12 km	26 km

Marathon

Table 7.21(a)	Peak mileage week microcycle for marathon: novice 4x					
Mon	Tues	Wed	Thurs	Fri	Sat	Sun
D/O	20 km	D/O	16 km	D/O	10 km	30 km

Table 7.21(b)	Peak mileage week microcycle for marathon: semi-competitive 5x					
Mon	Tues	Wed	Thurs	Fri	Sat	Sun
D/O	20 km	10 km	16 km	D/O	12 km	30 km

155

Table 7.21(c)	Peak mileage week microcycle for marathon: semi-competitive 6x					
Mon	Tues	Wed	Thurs	Fri	Sat	Sun
6 km	20 km	10 km	16 km	D/O	12 km	30 km

Table 7.21(d)	Peak mileage week microcycle for marathon: elite to elite + 6x					
Mon	Tues	Wed	Thurs	Fri	Sat	Sun
6 km	25 km	10 km	20 km	D/O	20 km	36 km

Section C: Percentage ranges

The tables in this section give the percentages used to calculate training distances based on:

- number of weeks of speedwork
- hard/easy week ratio (mesocycle)
- percentage of training volume increase
- race distance.

N.B. Ideally keep your training programmes between nine and 14 weeks, to avoid becoming overly fatigued.

Block A – four weeks' speedwork
Mesocycle: 2 hard weeks, 1 easy week

A = 7% training volume increase for a long race
B = 7% training volume increase for a short race
C = 10% training volume increase for a long race
D = 10% training volume increase for a short race
See table 7.22(a).

Key

Long race = over 3.5 hours
Short race = under 3.5 hours
H = hard week (high volume in base and high intensity in speedwork)
E = easy week

Table 7.22(a)	Block A – 4 weeks' speedwork. Mesocycle: 2 hard weeks, 1 easy week																							
	Base												Speed											
Week	1	2	3	4	5	6	7	8	9	10	11	12	13	14	15	16	17	18	19	20	21	22	23	24
	E	E	H	H	E	H	H	E	H	H	E	H	H	E	H	H	E	H	H	E	H	H	E	E
A	44	51	58	65	58	65	72	65	72	79	72	79	86	79	86	93	86	93	100	86	100	86	–	–
B	44	51	58	65	58	65	72	65	72	79	72	79	86	79	86	93	86	93	100	72	79	72	65	–
C	35	40	45	50	40	50	60	50	60	70	60	70	80	70	80	90	80	90	100	80	100	80	–	–
D	35	40	45	50	40	50	60	50	60	70	60	70	80	70	80	90	80	90	100	70	80	70	60	–

Mesocycle: 3 hard weeks, 1 easy week

E = 7% training volume increase for a long race
F = 7% training volume increase for a short race
G = 10% training volume increase for a long race
H = 10% training volume increase for a short race
See table 7.22(b).

Table 7.22(b)	Block A – 4 weeks' speedwork. Mesocycle: 3 hard weeks, 1 easy week																							
	Base																Speed							
Week	1	2	3	4	5	6	7	8	9	10	11	12	13	14	15	16	17	18	19	20	21	22	23	24
	E	H	E	H	H	H	E	H	H	H	E	H	H	H	E	H	H	H	E	H	H	H	E	E
E	44	51	44	51	56	58	51	58	65	72	58	72	79	86	72	86	93	93	100	93	100	93	–	–
F	44	51	44	51	56	58	51	58	65	72	58	72	79	86	72	86	93	93	100	86	79	72	65	–
G	40	45	40	45	40	55	45	60	70	80	60	80	85	90	80	90	95	90	100	95	100	90	–	–
H	40	45	40	45	40	55	45	60	70	80	60	80	85	90	80	90	95	90	100	90	80	70	60	–

Mesocycle: 4 hard weeks, 1 easy week

I = 7% training volume increase for a long race
J = 7% training volume increase for a short race
K = 10% training volume increase for a long race
L = 10% training volume increase for a short race
See table 7.22(c).

Table 7.22(c)	Block A – 4 weeks' speedwork. Mesocycle: 4 hard weeks, 1 easy week																							
	Base																Speed							
Week	1	2	3	4	5	6	7	8	9	10	11	12	13	14	15	16	17	18	19	20	21	22	23	24
	E	H	H	E	H	H	H	E	H	H	H	H	E	H	H	H	H	E	H	H	H	H	E	E
I	44	48	51	44	54	56	58	51	58	65	72	79	58	79	86	93	100	79	100	93	100	86	–	–
J	44	48	51	44	54	56	58	51	58	65	72	79	58	79	86	93	100	79	93	86	78	72	65	–
K	45	50	55	45	55	60	65	55	65	70	75	80	65	85	90	95	100	70	100	90	100	90	–	–
L	45	50	55	45	55	60	65	55	65	70	75	80	65	85	90	95	100	70	93	85	80	70	60	–

Block B – six weeks' speedwork

Mesocycle: 2 hard weeks, 1 easy week

A = 7% training volume increase for a long race
B = 7% training volume increase for a short race
C = 10% training volume increase for a long race
D = 10% training volume increase for a short race
See table 7.23(a).

Table 7.23(a)	Block B – 6 weeks' speedwork. Mesocycle: 2 hard weeks, 1 easy week																							
	Base																	Speed						
Week	1	2	3	4	5	6	7	8	9	10	11	12	13	14	15	16	17	18	19	20	21	22	23	24
	E	E	H	H	E	H	H	E	H	H	E	H	H	E	H	H	E	H	H	E	H	H	E	E
A	44	51	58	65	58	65	72	65	72	79	72	79	86	79	86	93	86	100	93	86	100	93	–	–
B	44	51	58	65	58	65	72	65	72	79	72	79	86	79	86	93	86	100	86	72	86	79	65	–
C	40	45	50	55	50	55	60	55	60	70	60	70	80	70	80	90	80	100	90	80	100	90	–	–
D	40	45	50	55	50	55	60	55	60	70	60	70	80	70	80	90	80	100	80	70	80	70	60	–

Mesocycle: 3 hard weeks, 1 easy week

E = 7% training volume increase for a long race
F = 7% training volume increase for a short race
G = 10% training volume increase for a long race
H = 10% training volume increase for a short race
See table 7.23(b).

Table 7.23(b)	Block B – 6 weeks' speedwork. Mesocycle: 3 hard weeks, 1 easy week																							
	Base																	Speed						
Week	1	2	3	4	5	6	7	8	9	10	11	12	13	14	15	16	17	18	19	20	21	22	23	24
	E	H	E	H	H	H	E	H	H	H	E	H	H	H	E	H	H	H	E	H	H	H	E	E
E	44	51	44	51	56	58	51	58	65	72	58	72	79	86	72	86	93	100	86	93	100	93	–	–
F	44	51	44	51	56	58	51	58	65	72	58	72	79	86	72	86	93	100	72	86	79	72	65	–
G	40	45	40	45	55	60	45	60	70	80	60	80	85	90	80	90	95	100	90	95	100	90	–	–
H	40	45	40	45	55	60	45	60	70	80	60	80	85	90	80	90	95	100	70	90	80	70	60	–

Mesocycle: 4 hard weeks, 1 easy week

I = 7% training volume increase for a long race
J = 7% training volume increase for a short race
K = 10% training volume increase for a long race
L = 10% training volume increase for a short race
See table 7.23(c).

Table 7.23(c)	Block B – 6 weeks' speedwork. Mesocycle: 4 hard weeks, 1 easy week																							
	Base															Speed								
Week	1	2	3	4	5	6	7	8	9	10	11	12	13	14	15	16	17	18	19	20	21	22	23	24
	E	H	H	E	H	H	H	E	H	H	H	H	E	H	H	H	H	E	H	H	H	H	E	E
I	44	48	51	44	54	56	58	51	58	65	72	79	58	79	86	93	100	79	100	93	100	93	–	–
J	44	48	51	44	54	56	58	51	58	65	72	79	58	79	86	93	100	79	93	86	78	72	65	–
K	45	50	55	45	55	60	65	55	65	70	75	80	65	85	90	95	100	70	100	90	100	90	–	–
L	45	50	55	45	55	60	65	55	65	70	75	80	65	85	90	95	100	70	90	85	80	70	60	–

Block C – eight weeks' speedwork

Mesocycle: 2 hard weeks, 1 easy week

A = 7% training volume increase for a long race
B = 7% training volume increase for a short race
C = 10% training volume increase for a long race
D = 10% training volume increase for a short race
See table 7.24(a).

Table 7.24(a)	Block C – 8 weeks' speedwork. Mesocycle: 2 hard weeks, 1 easy week																							
	Base															Speed								
Week	1	2	3	4	5	6	7	8	9	10	11	12	13	14	15	16	17	18	19	20	21	22	23	24
	E	E	H	H	E	H	H	E	H	H	E	H	H	E	H	H	E	H	H	E	H	H	E	E
A	51	58	65	72	65	72	79	72	79	86	79	86	93	86	93	100	79	93	100	79	100	86	–	–
B	51	58	65	72	65	72	79	72	79	86	79	86	93	86	93	100	72	93	86	72	79	72	65	–
C	40	45	50	60	50	60	70	60	70	80	70	80	90	80	90	100	80	90	100	80	100	80	–	–
D	40	45	50	60	50	60	70	60	70	80	70	80	90	80	90	100	80	90	80	70	80	70	60	–

Mesocycle: 3 hard weeks, 1 easy week

E = 7% training volume increase for a long race
F = 7% training volume increase for a short race
G = 10% training volume increase for a long race
H = 10% training volume increase for a short race
See table 7.24(b).

Table 7.24(b)	Block C – 8 weeks' speedwork. Mesocycle: 3 hard weeks, 1 easy week																							
	Base															Speed								
Week	1	2	3	4	5	6	7	8	9	10	11	12	13	14	15	16	17	18	19	20	21	22	23	24
	E	H	E	H	H	H	E	H	H	H	E	H	H	H	E	H	H	H	E	H	H	H	E	E
E		44	51	44	51	58	65	51	65	72	79	65	79	86	93	79	100	93	100	86	93	100	93	—	—
F		44	51	44	51	58	65	51	65	72	79	65	79	86	93	79	100	93	86	79	86	79	72	65	—
G		50	55	50	60	65	70	60	70	75	80	70	80	85	90	80	100	90	100	80	90	100	90	—	—
H		50	55	50	60	65	70	60	70	75	80	70	80	85	90	80	100	90	80	70	90	80	70	60	—

Mesocycle: 4 hard weeks, 1 easy week

I = 7% training volume increase for a long race
J = 7% training volume increase for a short race
K = 10% training volume increase for a long race
L = 10% training volume increase for a short race
See table 7.24(c).

Table 7.24(c)	Block C – 8 weeks' speedwork. Mesocycle: 4 hard weeks, 1 easy week																							
	Base															Speed								
Week	1	2	3	4	5	6	7	8	9	10	11	12	13	14	15	16	17	18	19	20	21	22	23	24
	E	H	H	E	H	H	H	E	H	H	H	H	E	H	H	H	H	E	H	H	H	H	E	E
I		44	48	51	44	54	56	58	51	58	65	72	79	58	79	86	93	100	86	100	93	100	93	—	—
J		44	48	51	44	54	56	58	51	58	65	72	79	58	79	86	93	100	86	93	86	79	72	65	—
K		45	50	55	45	55	60	65	55	65	70	75	80	65	85	90	95	100	80	100	90	100	90	—	—
L		45	50	55	45	55	60	65	55	65	70	75	80	65	85	90	95	100	70	85	80	75	70	60	—

Section D: Approximate mileage to duration conversion

Table 7.25(a)	Approximate mileage to duration conversion: cycling (based on 300 kph)
Distance (km)	Time (hr/min)
20	0:40
30	1:00
40	1:20
50	1:40
60	2:00
80	2:40
90	3
100	3:20
120	4:00
130	4:20
140	4:40
160	5:20
180	6:00
200	6:40

Table 7.25(b)	Approximate mileage to duration conversion: running (based on 5 min/km)
Distance (km)	Time (hr/min)
2	0:10
3	0:15
4	0:20
6	0:30
10	0:50
12	1:00
15	1:15
16	1:20
18	1:30
20	1:40
25	2:05
26	2:10
30	2:30
36	3:00

Table 7.25(c)	Approximate mileage to duration conversion: kayaking (based on 10 kph)
Distance (km)	Time (hr/min)
6	0:36
10	1:00
12	1:12
15	1:30
16	1:36
17	1:42
19	1:54
20	2:00
23	2:18
25	2:30
30	3:00
35	3:30
40	4:00
50	5:00

Table 7.25(d)	Approximate mileage to duration conversion: swimming (based on 60 m/min)
Distance (m)	Time (hr/min/sec)
250	0:04:10
500	0:08:20
750	0:12:20
1000	0:16:40
1250	0:20:50
1500	0:25:00
1750	0:29:10
2000	0:33:20
2250	0:37:30
2500	0:41:40
2750	0:45:50
3000	0:50:00
3250	0:54:10
3500	0:58:20
3800	1:03:20

Table 7.25(e)	Approximate mileage to duration conversion: rowing (based on 12 kph)
Distance (km)	Time (hr/min)
2	0:30
10	0:50
12	1:00
15	1:15
16	1:20
17	1:25
19	1:36
23	1:56

You can test yourself to make the duration conversions more accurate by the following method.

- Do a short workout at your average cruising pace (LSD)
- Record   1 Time: ....
              2 Distance: ....
- Use the calculations in appendix 8 to determine your speed.
              3 Speed: ....

You can use further calculations in appendix 8 to determine durations for all workouts. This will help to refine and personalise your training duration estimates.

How to use the blueprint to get your working programme

Design your own working programme template. You can use this, following the three steps below, to complete your weekly working programme.

1 Using your previous week's experience (and suggestions from your coach if you have one), you would put your calculated mileages from the relevant week in the blueprint into the working programme in *pencil.* Using pencil allows you to change the workout if you need to – remember, adjustments will be made as illness, fatigue, work commitments, etc. have an effect on your training.

2 As you complete each workout, write it down in pen over the top of the figures you have written in pencil, and then fill in the rest of the data. Filling in this data is very important because the questions in the working programme are similar to the sorts of questions a good coach would ask. How you answer provides a clear picture of how your training is going and how it might be modified to optimise performance.

Complete the questions in the performance analysis by circling the appropriate answers. This way you fill out all the specific information quickly and in a set order, which makes it easy to refer to. The circles also allow you to assess your training very quickly because they clearly show up patterns (good and bad) in training. Other relevant specifics (if required) can be filled out in the log book in the standard way.

3 Once you have completed your training week, complete the weekly summary. Look for patterns and errors that harm your training. Record these in the training notes. And look for ways to refine and improve your training. You won't find something every week, of course, but it may happen often enough to make a real difference in the way you train. Ways of picking up training faults and strengths are described in the next chapter, on training analysis. Once the working programme has been completed and summarised, it then becomes your log book. This is then used in conjunction with the blueprint to help you write and refine each week's new working programme.

Important points when using your training programme

1 Don't do every workout, every week, every month, regardless of how you feel. This will not work, and you will end up overtrained. Listen to your body. Remember the principles we have discussed so far in this book. You will probably miss 5 to 20 per cent of your workouts. This is normal, and you shouldn't worry about it. If you are missing more than 10 to 20 per cent of your workouts you may need to reassess how much training you have set yourself – it may be too much.

2 If you miss a workout, it is gone. Never try to 'bring it back', as this will destroy the balance of your programme and you may end up overtrained.

3 Don't develop 'accountancy mentality'. You should not try to balance your log book numbers.

4 Listen to your body!!

Racing logs

You should not only plan and log how you train, but also how you race. This means that after the race you can assess your plan and identify areas for improvement. Fig. 8.1 provides an example of a race plan and log analysis.

Refinement to the race plan: In my next race I need to relax more. Because of this I lost control and took too long to find my rhythm.
Refinement to the training plan: Based on the other responses, it appears I was uncomfortable with the waves, I need to practise this more in my next training programme.

Figure 8.1 Race plan and log analysis for swim leg of a triathlon	
Aspect of the race	Rating
1. Running beach start	Good
2. Dolphin dives first few waves	OK
3. Swim hard first 200 m	Good
4. Settle and try to relax	Poor
5. Get control of what needs to be done in the race plan without getting spooked	Poor
6. Find rhythm	Poor
7. Wave duck dives	OK
8. Set up drafting position	OK
9. Rounding the first buoy to go wide	Good
10. Long and strong to the second buoy	Good
11. Keep checking open-water navigation: swim straight	Good
12. On homeward leg use landmark sighting	Good
13. Kick final 200 m	Good
14. Swim until you touch twice	Good
15. Stand quickly and begin to remove wetsuit, then goggles, then swim cap	Good

PREPARING FOR RACE DAY

The importance of preparation

The alarm goes off: it's race day. There's the quiet drive in the dark to the race venue. There's no one out at that time of the morning on the rain-soaked streets. Everything is very still under the haze of streetlights, it's eerie. You manage to park the car, which is hard since the place is packed and you're running a little late. You open the car door and immediately feel the chill in the air. Your nerves start to jangle as you take your gear out of the back of the car, trying to hurry since you're late, while trying not to hurry and remain calm. As you make your way to the start there is that same eerie quiet as athletes, eyes glassed over, absorbed in their own thoughts, pass by and spectators look on, whispering under their breath. The closer you get to start time the more you feel the adrenaline pulse through your veins. There is energy and hype all around you. The time is drawing closer. A megaphone starts to boom out information that doesn't fully penetrate all the thoughts in your head. What does make it through the mental fog is that there are only five minutes to race start. Later, you hear two minutes. The air is heavy with a mixture of adrenaline, anxiety and fear. You struggle to relax, clear the extraneous thoughts from your head and get into the 'racing zone'. You see terror in the eyes of some of the athletes around you. Suddenly, without warning, the gun goes off and immediately everything is happening too fast. There's jostling and confusion, you feel the fear rise in your throat and desperately try to relax.

Welcome to the world of racing. Interestingly, a lot of the atmosphere and competition requirements of race day are not experienced until the moment they happen. This is because many athletes don't take the time to prepare properly for race day, or to adapt their training to the specific event. In the case of a triathlon they may not give much thought to whether it's a hilly or a flat course, to the possibility of a rough sea swim, to the requirements of a beach start to the swim that you have trained for 6 to 12 months for, for running into the transition area, finding your bike, putting on all your gear quickly and efficiently, and what you do in the first few minutes on the bike as you leave the transition area. All that seems to matter is how often you ride your bike, how many kilometres you do and how hard you are pushing yourself. However, without preparing for race day a lot of this training is a waste of energy.

For example, I've seen athletes do 108 km of swim training in a pool over 3 months, thinking the requirements to prepare for a 2 km sea swim involve the following: a 3km swim per session, backwards and forwards, in interval fashion rather than continuously, in fresh water, inside, without any waves, without a wetsuit, without anyone around them, following a black line (instead of open-water navigation), at faster than race pace. They believe that if they do this, they will be ready for the big day. Swimmers who usually swim 2 km in the pool in 30 minutes can end up taking 50 minutes in rough seas if they haven't practised for the conditions that they will encounter in the race. Pool swimming certainly has its place, but if you've never practised an open-water beach start, odds are you'll have a lousy start to your race.

Playing the game

A race result is based not only on how you train, but also on how you 'play the game'. Playing the game is just as important as all the training miles you work so hard at, so put some time into getting it right.

Always set a game plan for your race. Most people do all the training but forget the race plan. That is like a general training his soldiers for the physical elements of an upcoming battle, but going into battle without a battle plan. His army would be slaughtered. A race is like a battle; there are a series of steps. If each step is carried out flawlessly, you have a perfect race.

Here are some points that are worth thinking about before doing your big race.

Make a list of everything required in the race and train for them

Work out all the things that you will experience on race day. Your training should then show your body what will happen on the day (in small doses) and in the order in which they will occur.

For example, triathlon training should first show your body the disciplines of swimming, biking and running. Then show it the distances. Once your body knows this, show it all the details: the bike you'll ride, the gear you'll wear, what you'll eat and drink, and how much and how often. Finally, show your body the condi-

tions, the course, the weather conditions, the race hype, pressure and competition. Having experienced every detail of the event in training, your body should be able to precisely describe what will happen on race day. For example, it should be able to say that a triathlon starts with a swim, which will be at a certain pace, in a wetsuit, in the sea, with a lot of people beside it, over a certain distance and over a certain course. If your preparation is good enough, there won't be a single thing that happens on race day that your body hasn't experienced before, which makes it very hard to have a bad day.

A good race plan is like a surgical operation: efficient, clinical and precise. Fig. 9.1 provides an example of a training plan for racing the swim section of a triathlon.

Figure 9.1 Training plan for racing the swim section of a triathlon

Specifics: 1500 m, sea, beach start, surf
- Practise running beach start
- Practise dolphin dives
- Practise hard first 200 m
- Practise settling and trying to relax
- Practise getting control of what needs to be done in your race plan without getting spooked
- Practise finding rhythm
- Practise wave duck dives
- Practise drafting
- Practise surges
- Practise rounding the first buoy
- Practise long and strong to the second buoy
- Practise open water navigation
- Practise homeward leg landmark sighting
- Practise kicking final 200 m
- Practise swimming until you touch twice
- Practise standing quickly and beginning to remove wetsuit then goggles and swim cap

---

Practise on smaller races

Go to smaller 'like' events and practise your race plan so that you can work on each aspect in racing conditions and under pressure. You may feel that you had a successful event if you finally nailed the start, which had been a weak point in previous events. This allows you to modify and refine how you race. It usually is not about what placing you get, but rather about whether you executed your plan perfectly.

Learn the course

Make sure you train on the course before race day. This is easy if the race is in your home-town. If not, you might make one or two special trips late in your programme to check out the course, if the race is very important. If you can't do this, then turn up at the race a few days before if it's a 'biggie'. Alternatively, turn up a few hours before if it's not as important. Ride or drive the course and learn every detail. If someone were to ask you what the course is like, your answer should be: 'Have you got two hours, because that's how long it would take to tell you about it'. You should know it that well.

Think about it. If you did a 5 km running time trial over a course you know, you would perform better than if the same distance time trial was on a course you were unfamiliar with. You would know how to pace yourself, where you were and how to deal with the terrain. The idea is to make each race 'home turf' and there-fore give yourself 'home advantage'.

Set a plan for the course

Go over the course from landmark to landmark and work out how you will approach each part of the event. Work out where you can attack using your strengths, and where your weak-nesses are and where you will therefore need

to defend. Work out how you will do it. For example, an athlete in a cycle race may be thinking, 'Where can I attack my opposition on the bike? Where will I need to defend? Where do I need to be in the bunch going into a corner? What can I do coming out of that corner with the wind behind me?'

Use other people's experience

Talk to other experienced athletes or coaches who have raced on the course before about any other factors (e.g. wind conditions on the day), and to see if there is anything you've missed.

Set up your 'computer programme'

The idea here is that you manage and control the race by setting up all the tasks that need to be completed: no surprises means a smooth running race. This also helps you to correctly visualise the race. On race day, you then just run the computer programme (*see* fig. 9.2 for an example). Take a running race over rocky terrain. If you've been over the course and know it well, you'll know exactly where to put your feet for every step. Your competition will obviously struggle to keep up.

Here's an example of the importance of having such a detailed plan. In the Ironman run at Lake Taupo, New Zealand, at one point there is a choice of a steep climb up a hill on the footpath or a more gradual climb on the road. The obvious choice if you are running and want to make life easy is to run up the road. Running up the footpath is harder and will 'kill' your legs, which is not smart racing. When do you think most athletes decide which route to take? Yep, the moment they see it on race day. While this may not seem like much, there are tens and maybe even hundreds of decisions like that in

Figure 9.2 Example of the 'computer programme' for the transition area, pre-race for a triathlon

1 Enter transition area and set up bike (facing forwards, helmet upside on tri bars if not too many bikes, lay out bike and running gear on red towel on ground)
2 Go and get numbered
3 Come back to bike and set gear, cranks 3 o'clock and 9 o'clock, pump up tyres, put drink bottles in
4 Check tidal conditions for swim advantage
5 Check swim landmark for swim in
6 Check swim exits, note problems, take mental snapshot of transition from exit
7 Walk transition take mental snapshot of bike location from entrance
8 Walk to bike, counting rows and looking for landmarks (including red towel)
9 Note bike exit: mental snapshot and possible mishap areas
10 Check first 500 m of bike exit
11 Check bike entrance: mental snapshot and gear location
12 Note run exit and finish line
13 Put on wetsuit
14 Put on swim cap, goggles under cap
15 Stretch
16 Warm-up swim 5 min: 2-3 X 30 sec at race pace (if water cold, put wetsuit on and enter water at last minute)
17 Go to race start 5 min before start; keep warm

a race. If you are making every one of these decisions on the day as you experience them, you'll get probably 20 per cent of them wrong. You will have lost anywhere between two minutes and two hours, or even caused yourself to be unable to complete the race.

In summary, don't just train, make sure you are a master of 'playing the game'. There are only two reasons (excluding acts of God) for you to have a bad day: you either have a 'training surprise', which means something happened during the race that your body had not experienced in training, or you have a 'racing surprise', which means something happened during the race that you didn't have a plan for. There are very very few cases of straight out bad luck, almost always if you really go through it, they fall into one of the other two categories!

Training vs execution

Many athletes think that if they've done all the preparation, they're ready to go. However, that would be like setting up a sales presentation and never practising your delivery. You obviously need to do the preparation, but you also need to be able to execute the preparation on the day.

Once you get to race day, two things hold true:

1 You can't change your physiology – all the training has been done; you can only control how you use it.
2 You can't control what happens to you on the day and you may have some bad luck, but you can control how you handle it.

This means that being able to focus can have a huge effect on your final performance, no matter how well prepared you are physically. In many races, particularly the longer or high-pressure events, it's usually the head that lets you down, and part of the reason is that the head is often not nearly as well trained as the body. You should aim to control each 50 m of the course, one at a time. Imagine that each 50 m is one round of a boxing match where either you win or the course wins, then set about winning as many rounds as possible. The more rounds you win, the closer you get to the perfect race. What this boils down to is that there are two aspects to every event:

1 Attack: what you do to the event; and
2 Defence: what the event does to you.

Attack

Following are the components of attack.

The 50 m rule

The 50 m rule is about optimising every 50 metres: constantly looking for the shortest, fastest line. It's about looking for an opportunity to look after your legs on the hills, using the wind, avoiding the sun if you can, finding the smoothest bit of the road. There is no even ground: you are either gaining time/control on the course, or you are losing time/control of the course.

Urgency: every second counts

If you saved 15 seconds every five minutes, over the course of a $12^{1}/_{2}$ hour Ironman you would save a massive $37^{1}/_{2}$ minutes. To put this into perspective, the difference between Jo Lawn and third-placed Lisa Bentley in the 2003 New Zealand Ironman was a miniscule 71-hundredths of a second for each minute that went by.

The message here is that every single second counts. This does not mean that you get all uptight; it means that you want to achieve a level of relaxed urgency. You should be relaxed, but understand that you can't mess around at any point. For example, in a state of relaxed urgency on your bike, you would do what you need to do without ever stopping pedalling:

• If you want to have a drink, have a drink, but don't stop pedalling.
• If you want to eat, eat, but don't stop pedalling.
• If you want to throw up on your bike, no problem, but don't stop pedalling.

Rhythm

The better your rhythm, the faster you go. To give you the idea of just how important rhythm is, let's take the exhausting process of moving house as an example. When you start it's hard, and you move slowly. By lunchtime, you speed up and get into the groove; it feels easier. You have rhythm, and then you have a one-hour lunch break. Soon after starting back into it, you discover that it's really hard. You've broken rhythm and therefore lost momentum.

1 If you break rhythm it is hard to reacquire or get back 'in the groove'.
2 The more fatigued you are the harder it is to reacquire rhythm.

In Ironman, rhythm is defined as arm or leg turnover rate, which is stride rate, cadence or stroke rate. So, for example, if you keep stride rate, cadence or stroke rate as uniform as possible, you will have rhythm. This might mean focusing on keeping to a 85–90 rpm cadence on the bike. It might mean ensuring that you shorten your stride length going up the hills on the marathon to hold stride rate. Holding rhythm is enormously useful in retaining speed in the latter parts of an event.

Flatten the hills

Another thing to do is to flatten the hills. Just about every cyclist that rides up a hill 'over works' it, and might produce 350 Watts of effort/power. However, almost every rider will also 'under work' when they ride down the hill and only produce 150 Watts. Some even freewheel downhill, which means 0 Watts. These fluctuations in effort mean a slower overall time, so you need a strategy to reduce them as much as possible.

Using the cycling portion of an Ironman triathlon as an example, if you 'soft pedal' up the hills you will generate a lower wattage/effort and will therefore look after your legs. This helps to save energy/muscle glycogen for later in the event. You might lose 10 seconds on the hill, but you'll probably get 60 seconds back later in extra energy. You then work on the downhills. This doesn't mean that you go harder; you just ride at the effort you would use on the flat on the downhill. This will mean that you are riding faster than most people ride down a hill because they are taking a 'breather'. Often, you will make up the 15 seconds that you lost on the uphill on the downhill, so you lose nothing and still have more energy. This 'flattens the hills', helps with rhythm and often improves your time. The same applies to the wind – work the tailwind and don't overwork the headwind!

'Slack'

Before you work on going faster take out all the 'slack', or the 'dead time'. This means no freewheeling downhills, no freewheeling when drinking from a bottle, and taking out all the stoppage times if you can. Every moment should involve moving forward.

It's amazing how slack time adds up. To give you an example, let's say you aimed to compete in a 500 km cycling enduro. If someone took 20 hours to ride 500 km, which included a 10-minute stop every two hours, that's five minutes per hour. This seems reasonable, but equates to 100 minutes. This accounts for a loss of riding distance of 45 kilometres if they were riding at 27 kilometres an hour.

In an Ironman, you might freewheel 15 times on the bike for 30 seconds, which might cost you seconds each time. That's 225 seconds in total, or nearly 4 minutes. You might think this is no big deal. But then let's say your transitions weren't well practised and you lost 2 minutes in each one, which is not unusual. That's another 4 minutes. Then let's say that at each of the 21 aid stations in the marathon, you were a little relaxed and took 15 seconds longer than you needed. That's 315 seconds, or just

over 5 minutes. Let's also say that you stopped 3 times to go to the toilet, totalling 2 mins each from slowing down to stop to accelerating back up to your correct pace. That's 6 minutes. If we add all this 'slack' time up, it works out at 19 minutes wasted time! That's 19 minutes you could take off your time for little or no effort.

Take the shortest line

When an event is advertised, the organisers state the distance: a marathon, for example, is 42.195 km. However, this is only the distance in the centre of the course. Therefore, you have the ability to reduce this distance to some extent by taking 'shorter lines'. This means running the shortest distance at all times, for example running around the inside of a corner as opposed to the outside. So, if you're a smart marathon runner you never run 42.195 kilometres; you run 41.2 kilometres.

Nutrition

You need a good hydration and nutrition strategy to keep your energy levels topped up. This means you can save your 'on-board' energy more effectively, meaning a faster second half of the event due to not having to slow down as much due to fatigue. Chapter 12 discusses nutrition in more detail.

Effort

The golden number one rule of any time trial type event like triathlons, time trials in cycling and a lot of running races is to start at the effort level you can finish at. The more you keep your effort at the correct sustainable effort level instead of having fluctuations in effort, the better you will perform towards the end of the event. Constant pace wins the race!

Technique

Good technique means the ability to use your effort to better effect, producing a faster result for no extra physical effort. It is inevitable that you will fatigue towards the end of an event, but you can still control your form or technique. As you tire, you can deteriorate physically and technically. The dropping of technical ability compounds the fatigue effects, slowing you still further. Fortunately, if you understand how to control your technique, you can stop this area deteriorating and save yourself time.

Table 9.1 shows you how to bring all of these elements together and list everything you need to focus on for each 50 m in an event.

Defence

However good your attack strategies, you will also need to defend yourself against anything the event throws at you.

Staying on top: positivity

Have you noticed that if someone says something positive to you, you feel great and it fills you with energy. Conversely, someone can say something that psyches you right out, and within minutes you feel terrible and totally deflated. It is therefore pretty obvious that being negative to yourself is of absolutely no help during the event. Stay positive at all costs, pretend that you have a 'negativity radar' that makes you aware of your own negative thoughts and gets rid of them. It takes a lot of effort to keep this on track, but it is a must. You can be as negative as you like, but it has to be after the event!

Staying in the moment

Always focus completely on the 'now' (with a little thought for what is immediately next). If you do this, you will fully optimise this moment before working on the next one, following the 50 m at a time rule. Most people are worried by what will happen next, or annoyed about a problem that occurred in the past. I have seen situations where an athlete gets an accidental drafting penalty in an Ironman triathlon and

Table 9.1	Attack strategies for an Ironman
Nutrition	What? When?
Effort	• Am I starting at the pace I can finish at? • Is my pace as smooth and even as possible? • Am I using the right effort to complete this race as fast as possible? • Flatten the hills!
Slack	• Am I removing 'dead time', time I do not have to waste, freewheeling? Downhill? Cycling too gently with the wind? Transitions? • Am I maximising dead time?
Course use	• Am I taking the smoothest line? • Am I taking the shortest line? • Am I using the wind?
Technique	• Can I increase my power for the same effort?
Rhythm/relaxation	• Can I acquire rhythm, become a metronome? • Can I relax all non-used muscles, and used muscles between contractions?

then spends the rest of the event unable to let it go as it slowly destroys their day.

The most common and dangerous psychological problem in any endurance event is that athletes get halfway through the event and then decide what will happen next. They then react to this, usually with negative results. For example, during the event they may find that they don't feel as good as they did an hour ago. They then think, 'Well, if this is where I am right now, at this rate I will be exhausted in another hour'. They have decided what is going to happen next. They then think, 'I've trained so hard to get here and it's all coming apart at the seams, I'll be walking in less than an hour and I'll have to walk 20 km. It's all falling apart.' They are now reacting to what they think is going to happen.

Instead, you should focus on what you need to do to rectify the situation now and focus on this alone. Forget about where that might lead, because you probably don't know and focusing on a perceived negative that might not happen will not help you in any way.

It's just your turn

We all dream of the perfect race, the one where nothing goes wrong. Unfortunately, all endurance events are fraught with potential problems. You might have the perfect day, but it's unlikely. At some point something is going to go wrong. Mentally prepare for this.

At this point, most athletes lose their composure, and fall into a negative spiral. You need to remember being 'blindsided' by a problem happens to just about everyone at some point, it's just that right now it happens to be your turn! Understand that what is happening to you is not unusual, and that how you react to your bad moment compared with how someone else reacts to their bad moment will define the race.

I remember preparing my best and hardest for one Ironman that I did. 70 km into the bike ride I broke a 'roller' in my chain and my chain jumped out of gear every second pedal stroke for the next 110 km. I was beside myself with rage; at one point with 30 km to go I got off my bike, gave up and threw my bike into a ditch! I thought, 'I'm in the middle of nowhere, no one is going to pick me up anytime soon,' and so thought I'd get back on my bike, ride back to town and give up. I then thought, 'If I'm riding back into town I may as well race, because if my chain breaks now, big deal!" As I arrived at T2 I thought, 'I'm here now, I may as well do the marathon.' So I ran out onto the marathon and did the run of my life, achieving the time I had set as a goal and qualifying for the Kona World Champs!

Was it the perfect day? No! Could I have gone faster? Sure but I didn't. What I did do was stay mentally tough in my crisis moment and still hang on to pull the result out of the bag. So, if something goes wrong, realise that it's just your turn, focus on fixing the problem instead of whining about it and you'll be surprised what you can do.

Disassociation

If you slam your fingers in a car door as you get out of the car and then the car rolls backwards onto your leg and breaks it, you will quickly forget your sore fingers because your leg hurts so much. It's interesting that you have such exceptional mind control because your fingers should still be hurting; however, you can only think one thought at a time and you feel what you focus on. To take a less extreme example, you wake up in the morning 'sick as a dog' and think that there is no way you could manage getting through a working day. However, once you're at work you don't feel as sick. This is because you have something else to think about.

Pain is 40 per cent physiological and 60 per cent mental interpretation, which means that to some extent you can control any pain you experience during the event. If you do start to experience pain, you need to focus on something else. What do you focus on? The 50 m rule and every second counts. If you focus on those two things you don't have time to think about anything else.

Suffocation (two pink hippos)

The next defence trick is suffocation. Now suffocation is based on what I call two pink hippos. There are two pink hippos in a duckpond surrounded by lily pads, frogs and big orange goldfish, with long reeds all around the pond and nicely mown grass in the background. Despite the fact that we are discussing high-performance racing, two pink hippos wallowing in water surrounded by ducks is probably what you are thinking about.

The crucial point is that you can only hold one conscious thought in your head at any one time. You can't think two conscious thoughts at the same time. You can think about doing your event or pink hippos (or pink hippos doing your event) but you can't think about pink hippos *and* your event at the same time.

So, if the little voice in the back of your head says something like: 'it's such a long way to go; your knees are starting to hurt; you won't make it; you've been in this situation before and you had trouble, it's going to be the same again here,' you have to suffocate the thought. You can do this by stating a positive thought that constructively fixes the present problem, keeps your mind off the negative thinking and keeps your morale up. For example: 'Getting angry or disheartened right now doesn't fix anything. I need to forget everything else and work out how to fix the situation right now.'

Once you have the answer, repeat it to yourself over and over in your head. It must be a short, succinct answer to the problem at hand.

For example, if you have had a drop in energy you would say something like 'Get to the next aid station and get some energy,' over and over for 30 seconds to a minute to suffocate the negative thought. You can't think 'I'm tired' and 'Get to the next aid station and get some energy' at the same time, so make sure it's the positive thought in your head!

Coach yourself

Imagine you cloned yourself. One of you is doing an event and the other is a coach watching you as you go around the course. The coach is watching with another person, who we'll call Bob. Every time you go past, Bob shouts in your ear the little negative thoughts that drift through people's heads when they are doing an endurance event. How would you the coach react to Bob shouting these negative comments at you the athlete? You would be furious and would defend 'you' the athlete very strongly, saying that it's hard enough doing the event without having all the negative stuff shouted at you as well.

If you defend you the athlete strongly when you are their coach, why wouldn't you defend yourself any differently against those little negative thoughts during an event anyway? Negativity can spread like a virus in your thinking during an event and pull you down. Keep coaching yourself, encouraging yourself and driving yourself.

The importance of positivity

An athlete with a head full of negativity will almost always be beaten by a positive athlete if they are of a similar ability. The top of any sport is all about pressure. Pressure in part tests whether or not you are able to maintain a positive frame of mind for the whole duration of the event.

Rewards

At some point during an endurance event when the pain gets tough you will do a calculation in terms of the reward versus the pain. At this point either the pain will be higher than the reward and your event will fall to pieces, or the reward is greater than the pain and you will carry on regardless.

So, what motivation could you put in place to ensure that you got the job done? Think of something so powerful that when you get to the point where you have to do the calculation the reward is so strong that the pain never wins. For example:

- If you were doing it in memory of some one very dear to you, would you let them down?
- If you could have £1 million free every year for the rest of your life, could you finish the event?

It doesn't matter what it is, but if you can find something that seriously emotionally charges you it will increase your drive to the point where you will never give up.

You do have to be a little careful with this technique in that you still have to know when you need to stop because you are doing yourself harm. If you then miss the goal you can end up pretty depressed, so use this tool carefully.

Gang up

We know that people struggle when they are alone. What if you have some friends on their bikes while you're running, stopping and cheering you as you go past, then riding further down the road and again cheering as you go past? It's not you against the event anymore, it's you and your gang against the event! This is particularly useful in the second half of an event.

Be a perfectionist

Many top performers have a different way of looking at the world from the rest of us. They are perfectionists more than they are competitors. They want to win, but the way in which they go about achieving this is different from most of us. They are more internally focused than external; in other words, they are more focused on the process than the outcome. Rather than focusing on one aspect of performance (such as time or distance, winning gold or smashing a world record), their focus is on perfection in all the skills that create the performance. They then combine every element to create the ultimate result.

The focus and drive of these competitors is primarily internal: they still want to win, but what they focus on is different. This highlights a key point: there is a big difference between the goal and what you focus on. The goal is the outcome, it is not how you get there. Focus on the process, win each task that you need to perform and let the outcome take care of itself.

THE COACH

10

The value of the coach

If you possibly can, get a coach or experienced athlete to help you with your training, even if it is just now and again. Most experienced athletes and coaches are only too happy to share their knowledge. Coaching is an invaluable aid. The experience and knowledge of a good coach allows you to progress faster because pitfalls and mistakes are avoided. They also provide an objective opinion on your training, and are very good for motivation as they tend to push you to greater efforts when required. Good technique can also be taught by the coach, which can have a huge effect on performance, and his/her advice on the choice of equipment and its set-up can significantly help performance.

The relationship between athlete and coach

Communication is vital between the coach and the athlete and the communication must always be two-way! The coach is a guide and consultant, not a dictator. He or she needs to know how the athlete is feeling and responding to training. This requires a thorough dialogue. It is also important to know whether the athlete is 'picking up' aspects of training which may require work: for example, in rowing this may include things like slide control, movement of the boat at the catch, complete unity of the crew in leg drive.

When writing the next training programme

the coach should use data from previous training logs and input from the athlete. (Inexperienced athletes will obviously need to rely more on the coach's experience than experienced athletes.)

The key to good coaching is the coach's knowledge of the sport, his/her experience, the ability to relate to many personality types, an understanding of how to get the most out of an athlete, communication with the athlete based on equality, the desire and need to continue learning, and a willingness always to put the athlete's welfare first.

Level of coach involvement

Coaching an inexperienced athlete requires a high level of coach involvement. The coach needs to explain the hows and whys of training, including the reason it is structured the way it is. In this way, the athlete will gain a better understanding of training and will be able to have a greater input into the programme.

Initially, the coach is a benevolent dictator when it comes to training. As the athlete's training knowledge increases, however, and they become more self-sufficient, the coach takes on more of a consultancy role, more concerned with fine-tuning than designing the programme entirely.

A coach should always accept that they can learn from the athlete, and there is a philosophy which suggests the coach has done a good job if the athlete surpasses the achievements of the coach (this makes it tough if you are coached by an Olympic champion!).

Responsibilities of the athlete, coach and administrator

The athlete's responsibilities

- To have fun
- To have self-discipline, dedication and self-motivation
- To learn to understand his/her own training
- To be realistic
- To respect and listen to the coach/administrators
- To set his/her own goals (short and long-term)
- To be able to take disappointments
- To have humility when successful
- To take full responsibility for his/her own performance
- To be professional in dealing with coaches, administrators, the public, the media and sponsors.

The coach's responsibilities

- To encourage the athlete
- To ensure the athlete's welfare always comes first
- To ensure the goals set are primarily the athlete's goals
- Not to push the athlete too hard
- To let the athlete make her/his own decisions
- To help the athlete's training in every way possible
- To make sure the athlete develops athletically and socially
- To ensure the athlete learns from and understands her/his training
- To make sure the athlete enjoys training
- To teach and allow the athlete self-sufficiency.

The administrator's responsibilities

- To make sure the athlete's (and coach's) welfare comes first
- To look after the best interests of the sport
- To ensure the athlete is freed from internal politics and administration and is able to train freely
- To ensure administration is effective and set up to help the athlete and coach
- To ensure the athlete can train and compete without administrative interference
- To encourage the athlete
- To provide opportunities that the athlete is unable to create for her/himself
- To provide organisational and developmental support for the athlete and coach
- To set up racing, training and coaching at the best times for the athlete
- To help raise funds for the athlete
- To ensure the sport's image is a positive one that provides plenty of opportunities for participation and enjoyment.

Coaching young athletes

Don't bury a young athlete under a mountain of work. A critical aspect of coaching young athletes is an understanding of their athletic development. It is important to realise that improvement will take place over many seasons and that the first few years of an athlete's career are somewhat akin to an apprenticeship.

The emphasis early on should be on fun and learning, not on results. Let the young athlete gain some experience and establish a training pattern. Don't burden them with expectations of success and records. Let them gain an understanding of their training and how it will develop them as an athlete.

Success in endurance sports takes many years to achieve at the highest level, and trying to 'bring on' a young athlete too soon may see them lose interest in the sport long before they have had a chance to enjoy all the sport has to offer (and any success that may have come their way). Too many coaches seem prepared to sacrifice an athlete's long-term prospects and short-term enjoyment for the sake of records and championships that may mean more to the coach than the athlete. With young athletes it can be tempting to create a junior champion through sheer volume of training. This often amounts to a coach abusing his/her power and feeding his/her ego, both at the expense of the athlete.

Fun and learning – those are the twin pillars upon which young athletes should be supported.

THE ENVIRONMENT – ALTITUDE, HEAT, COLD AND TRAVEL

11

You may have had a perfect training build-up, and you may be at the absolute peak of your performance potential, but a mistake in how you acclimatise to the racing climate or travel to the race venue can mean all your good preparatory work is wasted. It is very important, therefore, that you understand how climate and travel can disrupt performance. Acclimatisation can be defined as physiological compensation to environmental stress over a period of time.

Altitude training

Many athletes use altitude training as a way of getting that extra edge in terms of performance enhancement. It has been a highly controversial and contested area for quite a number of years and the official line remains: 'we cannot say unequivocally whether altitude training leads to improvements in sea level performance.'

Nevertheless, there is a large body of anecdotal evidence, combined with significant scientific research, showing that key physical and biochemical 'performance lifters' respond positively to altitude training.

What is altitude all about?

The most basic way to think about the effect of altitude is to imagine 'squashed air'! Air is more compressed near the earth's surface because there is a heavy blanket of atmosphere sitting on top of it. If you go to higher altitudes there is less atmosphere sitting above you so the weight of the air is less, which means it is less compressed and therefore there is less air in a given area. This explains why it is often said that the air is thinner at altitude.

One of the results of high altitude is that there are less oxygen molecules present. At the summit of Mount Everest there is only 30 per cent of the oxygen available at sea level, which means a resting heart rate of 64 has to work at double the rate (123 beats/min) to supply oxygen and this is still not enough! An un-acclimatised person taken from sea level directly to the summit of Mount Everest would pass out in about three minutes and die in roughly 10 minutes from lack of oxygen!

When there is less oxygen, it affects the function of the haemoglobin (the part of blood that transports oxygen from the lungs to the muscles). This means that the working muscles don't function as well during exercise because they don't receive as much oxygen.

Aerobic ability begins to decline at approximately 1524 metres (5000 feet) above sea level. Initially, a 3 percent decrease in aerobic ability occurs every 300 metres (1000 feet). At higher altitudes, however, the rate of decrease is much greater; for example, exercising at 3050 metres (10,000 feet) is more than twice as difficult as exercising at 1500 metres (5000 feet) (*see* table 11.1). Very simply, at altitude there is a reduction in aerobic ability. This

Table 11.1	Effect of altitude on aerobic ability
Altitude	Aerobic ability
0 m	100%
1,976 m (6,500 ft)	90%
3,286 m (14,100 ft)	75%
6,992 m (23,000 ft)	50%

in turn reduces performance in endurance sports.

Performance changes at altitude

- 100–400 m: enhanced 1 to 2 per cent
- 3,000 m steeplechase to 5,000 m: impaired by 5 to 6 per cent
- 10,000 m to marathon: impaired 6 to 7 per cent

The body adapts to altitude stress by increasing haemoglobin and red blood cell production. At 4,500 metres red blood cell levels increase by 20 per cent in three to four weeks. This means the oxygen-carrying capacity is increased and more oxygen theoretically gets to the muscles. Performance potential at that altitude is then increased from the initial unadapted state. If you return to sea level after altitude adaptation, the adaptation remains briefly, allowing a higher oxygen carrying capacity in the blood and theoretically a level of performance that could not have been achieved if you had stayed at sea level.

Ways of generating the same effect unnaturally include what is known as 'blood doping' (an infusion of the athlete's own blood or someone else's back into his/her body). This has the effect of supplying more red blood cells, which means a higher oxygen-carrying capacity. There is also a drug called EPO (erythropoietin) which is used (illegally) by some endurance athletes because it increases red blood cell levels. Unfortunately for those athletes, it also increases

their chance of a heart attack as the increased blood cell levels thicken the blood to the point where the heart becomes overloaded and cannot pump it adequately.

Natural altitude training appears to give an improvement of approximately 0.5 per cent but this improvement is not as big as the 'hype' purports it to be. Of course, we shouldn't forget that an average difference of 0.5 per cent or less exists between gold and silver medallists at an Olympic games (*see* table 11.2). The gains don't have to be that big!

How to train at altitude

There are several different ways to approach altitude training. The main two methods are:

- Live High Train High – traditional altitude training
- Live High Train Low – this comes in several forms:

    Location based – Living in a training location at altitude but moving to areas at lower altitudes to train.

    Nitrogen houses – Living in a house that is sealed and pumped with air containing reduced amounts of oxygen. This was initially set up in Finland, where they have no geographical regions of high altitude. The nitrogen house is a series of well-furnished apartments where the altitude equivalent is approximately 2000 to 3000m (6560 to 9840

Table 11.2	Differences in performance at the 2000 Olympics Men's 10,000 m	
Difference	%	
1st & 2nd	0.005	
1st & 3rd	0.03	
1st & 4th	0.08	

feet). In several countries, elite athletes have nitrogen apartments within their homes where they spend eight to 18 hours a day. The ventilation system pulls in ambient air (20.93 per cent oxygen and 79 per cent nitrogen) and adds nitrogen gas to create air that is reduced in oxygen and higher in nitrogen (15.3 per cent oxygen and 84.7 per cent nitrogen)

Altitude tents and rooms – These are sealed tents or rooms that have a dial controlling 'altitude' within them. They use an oxygen filtering membrane that reduces the oxygen content from the air outside and pumps it into the living area, creating 'altitudes' of up to 4000meters (14000 feet). These can be quite claustrophobic and small.

Intermittent hypoxic exposure – This technique involves breathing into a mask for short periods at a time. This can be used to create exposure to altitude at rest or to create altitude adaptation during exercise. Currently, it is not clear whether this can serve as an effective alternative to four or more weeks of altitude exposure.

I believe that the location-based live high train low is the most effective strategy for altitude training However, you should make sure that you go to a well-serviced location. Altitude-training camps are still very popular and a lot of top coaches swear by them.

How often should the strategy be used?

One option is to go to altitude twice each year. Frank Dick, a top training expert for the British Athletics Federation, suggested that athletes should spend three weeks at a time at altitude. This would be long enough to get the 'altitude effect' but short enough so overall fitness didn't deteriorate. Each stay would be at approximately 2000 m. The first stay would be at the end of the off-season/early pre-season after winter training. The second would be during the final preparation for your major event and peak competition. You could live high and train low all the time, but I have not seen enough evidence to say whether the effect is greater than the twice a year strategy.

Live high train high traditional altitude training camps for sea level residents:

How high?

The optimal altitude in which to live appears to be somewhere between 2100 metres (6898 feet) and 2500 metres (8200 feet). Locations below 2100 metres may not be high enough to stimulate red blood cell production, whereas living above 2500 metres may lead to training recovery problems.

How long do you need to stay at altitude to gain the benefits?

The recommended minimum stay is four to six weeks at altitude.

How do you structure training?

An acclimatisation period of one week followed by the altitude training (two to four weeks) seems to be most common.

Training Volume:

Initially reduce sea level training volume by 10 to 20 per cent. Gradually increase the training volume by 3 per cent to 5 per cent per week. Altitude experienced athletes may be able to reach normal sea level training volumes by the end of the training period.

Training Intensity/Pace:

Interval training must be at a slower pace than when at sea level. This is very individualised but the basic guideline is a reduction of 5 to 7 per cent. Gradually increase the pace by around 1 – 2 per cent per week over the duration of the altitude training.

Rest Periods Between Efforts:

The duration of the interval training rest period between efforts must be longer. Once again, this is highly individualised but a basic guideline is to double the time of rest between intervals. Gradually adjust this by decreasing the rest by 2 or 3 per cent per week over the training period. It has been noted that athletes that regularly go to altitude can reduce their rest periods by up to 25 per cent per week over a 5-week period.

Note: An athlete's ability to cope with altitude is highly varied. These are guidelines only and should be experimented with and based on individual tolerances.

What is the timing for return to sea level for competition?

The optimal timing for return to sea level is once again highly individualised. Therefore, the optimal schedule should be determined through experimentation and training build-ups prior to the championship event. It seems that the longer the event, the longer the time period between returning from altitude and the key competition.

What is the duration of altitude training effects?

There is an anecdotal consensus that the altitude training effect lasts approximately two or three weeks, although others are convinced that they can last as long as two months. The recommendation is that you experiment.

Live high train high permanent altitude residents (over 1500 m)

Here are some considerations for permanent altitude residents:

Sea-level training before major competition

Most of the year is spent at altitude but four to six weeks before a major competition the athlete comes down to sea level for six weeks. Alternating between sea level and altitude might also be an effective option.

Replicating sea-level training

You cannot expect to replicate sea level training at altitude – particularly in terms of speed. Some coaches use the following methods to get around this:

- *Shorter than sea level intervals* e.g. if the sea level workout is 6 x 1600 m, the workouts might be broken into 200 m or 400 m efforts to allow the athlete to accurately replicate race pace efforts.
- *Train at lower altitudes* A 45 minute drive from Flagstaff, Arizona – 2165 m (7100 feet) is Camp Verde – 910 m (2985 feet). This is an example of a location that would allow you to live high and train low.
- *Downhill running* Another way to retain sea level speed is to do downhill running workouts on a 5 – 7 per cent downhill grade on a smooth grassy surface.
- *Supplemental Oxygen* Some athletes use supplemental oxygen during speed training to allow them to perform at sea level capacity.

Live high train low

Live high train low usually involves:

- living on the side of a mountain
- a nitrogen house
- an altitude tent
- Intermittent Hypoxic Exposure (resting or exercise).

Although most experts agree that this is the most effective system, there is not a lot of data on this method of altitude exposure. The key considerations of live high train low are that you need to spend at least eight to 10 hours

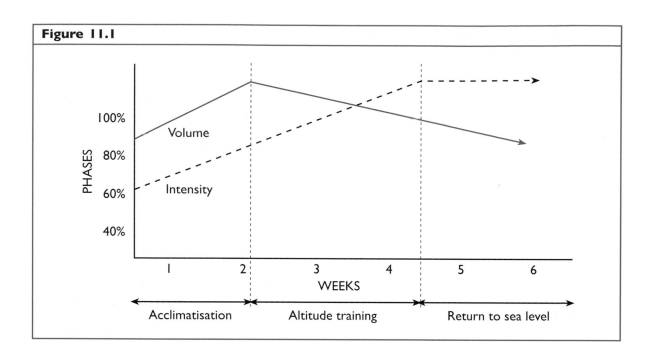

Figure 11.1

a day at 'altitude' and should either do this permanently or in periods of four to six weeks.

The altitude training phases

Phase One: Preparation phase

Athletes complete a health exam to determine their health status before going to altitude. Get blood tests six weeks and two weeks before you go, looking particularly at:

- ferritin (iron stores)
- iron
- baseline haemoglobin levels
- full blood count
- hematocrit (the volume of red blood cells per unit of blood)

Any deficiencies need to be addressed so that altitude training has its full effect. Foods rich in iron are an important part of the pre-altitude dietary plan. Low levels of iron stores can mean that the athlete may become sick soon after their arrival at altitude. The importance of B12

and folic acid in the production of red blood cells is also often overlooked.

The last seven to 10 days of sea-level training should be at low intensity. High intensity training and competition require extra recovery and this may impair acclimatisation.

Phase Two: Acclimatisation

There is a gradual acclimatisation over four to seven days, where the training is primarily aerobic. On the first day at altitude, training should only be very light and during this phase, no high-intensity training should be attempted. Exposure to a lot of open-air activity will help to promote acclimatisation. Most athletes train too hard at this stage, so take care that initial workouts are not too exhausting. Focus should be on long runs at easy to moderate intensity. Sea-level training volume is initially decreased to about 20 per cent, which is gradually increased back to 100 per cent through this phase.

Going to altitude – what will it be like?

The first two days of altitude training create no real problems other than shortness of breath. In the following days the athlete begins to feel very tired. A drop of 15 per cent in VO_2max may occur on the second day after arriving at 2200 metres. This is the time to be careful. It is easy to overtrain and damage your build-up. It is a good idea, therefore, to lower training intensity and volume during this period, and then to gradually build training levels back up.

On arrival at altitude

1. Don't just sit around during the first few days! Light exercise stimulates breathing and circulation, slightly quickening your adjustment. Train very lightly during the first few days.
2. Even if you have trouble sleeping, get plenty of rest.
3. You may want to use a humidifier to help combat the dry air at altitude.
4. Eat smaller meals but more frequently, since digestion can be difficult at altitude. Emphasise carbohydrates for recovery.
5. Avoid alcohol in the first three days at altitude and drink plenty of electrolyte drinks.
6. Susceptibility to infection is greater when at altitude. Good nutrition and proper adaptation to altitude can reduce the risk of illness. Athletes suffering from asthma may have more difficulty acclimatising.
7. Be prepared for sudden weather and temperature changes – these are often more extreme at altitude.
8. Dehydration seems to be amplified when training at altitude, so it is particularly important that you consume large quantities of electrolyte fluid before, during and after workouts. Weight should be checked before and after workouts and any weight loss should be overcome by adequate hydration. If weight loss has occurred through a workout, try to drink more the next time.

Phase Three: Altitude Training

With the initial acclimatisation period over, the athletes now embark on their altitude training in earnest. Over this period, training volume should build up over the first weeks and then taper back for the final week. For example, an eight-week altitude programme for elite male marathon runners starts at 80 km per week (50 miles), works up to 225 km (140 miles) per week by the fourth week and then tapers back to 70 km (43 miles) by the final week. Aerobic workouts are carried out at a slower pace – two to three minutes slower per 10,000 metres. The goal is to match sea level intensity (heart rate) as opposed to pace for aerobic and anaerobic efforts. Interval workouts are gradually added but the pace must be slower at altitude. For example, 4 x 1600 m at 4:40 pace would start at 5:00 at altitude and gradually reduce by approximately five seconds per week over the duration of a four- or five-week altitude period. There may be two loading phases (seven – 10 days each) followed each time by a regeneration phase of two or three days. The first loading phase is primarily intended for volume increase whereas the second loading phase focuses on increasing intensity.

Phase Four: Return to sea level

The first four to five days are devoted to recovery and reestablishment of a normal sea-level training pattern. The timing of your return to sea level in preparation for a race varies considerably for each individual. The recommendation is to try the following schedules:

- return one to two days prior to competition
- return approximately seven days prior to competition

- return approximately 10 days prior to competition

Opinions vary on the issue of timing the return to sea level. While some believe that marathon runners seem to achieve the best results seven to 10 days prior to returning from altitude, others think that athletes competing in the 5000 m and 10,000 m should return to sea level three weeks prior to a major competition. Most perform well after six to eight days at sea level. Athletes engage in more moderate training at this time, covering both aerobic and anaerobic training. Anaerobic 'leg turnover' intervals are done typically near the end of the re-acclimatisation phase. The beneficial effects of altitude training can last for approximately two weeks to one month after return to sea level, according to elite coaches that use altitude regularly.

Heart rate monitors and altitude

Heart rate monitors are very useful for avoiding training errors at altitude. Uses include:

1 Measuring degree of adaptation to altitude

In the first few hours at altitude, heart rate will drop. After this it will begin to rise. At 2,000 metres your heart rate will be about 10 per cent above your sea-level heart rate. At 4,500 metres, it will be about 50 per cent higher (until you begin to acclimatise). As you acclimatise, resting and training heart rates will return to normal, or even lower. At this point, acclimatisation is complete. By measuring the time it takes (i.e. the number of days) for both resting and training heart rates to return to sea-level rates, the length of adaptation can be calculated.

2 Matching altitude and sea-level intensities

It is easy to overdo initial training at altitude. The tendency is to push too hard because you are going so slowly (you may be faster on the bike, however, because of the reduction in air resistance). By using your heart rate monitor you can train at the same intensities that you would at sea level, without succumbing to the desire to increase your speed. (For example, an athlete running at altitude at his/her usual intensity will be performing at a slower pace due to the 'thin' air's effects on aerobic ability.) Once adaptation has taken place, training workloads similar to those carried out at sea level will be possible.

3 Setting correct rest periods between intervals

If you are doing speedwork at altitude, particularly intervals, rest periods need to be longer because recovery takes longer. To ensure your rest periods are not too short (or too long), make sure you don't begin exercising until your heart rate has dropped the same amount it would at sea level (40 to 60 bpm for most athletes). During the adaptation phase it will take longer for your heart rate to drop than it would at sea level at the same intensity.

Speedwork and altitude

Speedwork is affected during adaptation to altitude and, depending on the altitude, this may continue. For a distance runner, for example, speed is slower compared to similar intensities at sea level. This means the cardiovascular effect of training is the same, but the muscular and biomechanical effects are different.

Here are some guidelines for speedwork at altitude:

1. Give yourself enough time to adapt initially before engaging in speedwork.
2. Try to match your sea-level *intensity* (heart rate) to avoid overtraining. If you run at the *pace* you run at sea level your training will be too intense. Also, try doing shorter intervals at the correct pace but make sure that they are of a length that will not have too much of an

impact on your heart rate (e.g. 15 x 30 seconds at race pace with rest to recovery in between).

3. Do more hill efforts to counter the possible deterioration of strength endurance.

4. At altitude, 'Ramp' your pace over a period of weeks to give yourself enough time to adapt.

5. Increase the rest periods between efforts to allow adequate recovery and maximise the quality of your efforts. Gradually decrease them as you adapt to the altitude.

Competing at altitude

Competing at 1500 – 2000 m

The minimum acclimatisation period is 10 days (plus a taper period). As you will see in the information already provided, there is an anecdotal consensus that four to six weeks is probably more appropriate.

What if you can't achieve this?

If you do not have enough time to acclimatise, compete within 24 hours of arriving at altitude (essentially, the sooner the better) for a one-day event. The cumulative effects of altitude will not be fully felt immediately but performance will be lower than usual due to lack of time for adaptation. This is by no means the best way to do things, but it is better than the tiredness you will feel within 24–48 hours, as your body fatigues and starts the adaptation process.

Competing at above 2000 m

The worst time to compete is within one to three days after arrival at altitude. The answer here is that you *need* to acclimatise (seven to ten days minimum). Acute mountain sickness (common above 2100 m) usually occurs in the first 24 hours and subsides after 72 hours.

Note: For competitions lasting more than one day at altitude (under *and* over 2000 m), allow at least the minimum acclimatisation period.

Variations between preparing for racing at altitude and at sea level

1 Racing at altitude

You must do speedwork at altitude in order to adapt to racing in 'thin' air. During a four-to

Table 11.3	Altitude training programme used by Norweigan athletes, 2000 Winter Olympics (Salt Lake City)	
Phase	Duration	Objectives
One	14 days Nitrogen House – Norway 16 hours per day at 2700 m (8855 ft) Train 470 m (1540 ft)	acclimatise train in a normal O_2 environment
Two	14 days Live at 2500 m (8200 ft) – Utah Train at 1670 m to 1793 m (5480 – 5880 ft)	adjust to time zone build altitude ability train at competition-specific altitude
Three	16 days Live at 1700 m (5575 ft) – Utah Train at 1670 m to 1793 m (5480 – 5880 ft)	be close to competition venue live and train at competition-specific altitude

Environmental factors and acclimatisation time before a race

Example 1:
Travel: Cross 4 time zones, travelling westward (add 18 hr or 0.75 of a day per time zone)
Altitude: 2,000 m
Temperature: 10°

Environmental factor	Acclimatisation (before taper)		
	Minimum	Acceptable	Optimal
Travel	0	2–3 days	3+ days
Altitude	0	7–10 days	3 weeks or stepped adaptation (4–6 weeks)
Temperature	0	0	0

Total acclimatisation time (taking the environmental factor that requires the greatest acclimatisation time) means arrival at race venue (no. of days before the race):

Minimum: 0 days
Acceptable: 7–10 days
Optimal: 4–6 weeks

Example 2:
Travel: Cross 9 time zones, travelling eastward (add 24 hr or one day per time zone)
Altitude: 500 m
Temperature: 27°C

Environmental factor	Acclimatisation (before taper)		
	Minimum	Acceptable	Optimal
Travel	0	7–9 days	9–14 days
Altitude	0	0	0
Temperature	0	7–10 days	10–21 days

Total acclimatisation time (taking the environmental factor that requires the greatest acclimatisation time) means arrival at race venue (no. of days before the race):

Minimum: 0 days
Acceptable: 10 days
Optimal: 21 days

Note: Acclimatisation time does not include taper, which is a recovery from training period, not a time for adaptation to altitude, heat or a new time zone. If, for example, the time required to adapt to a new climate is 7–10 days and the taper period is 5 days, you should arrive there 10 + 5 days (acclimatisation plus taper) before competition.

SPORTS NUTRITION, RACE REHYDRATION AND REFUELLING

12

Shona Goldsbury

Shona Goldsbury (Dip HSc, RD) is a consultant dietitian specialising in sports nutrition. She was one of the first practitioners to be employed in the fitness industry in New Zealand in the mid 1980s, and now runs her own private practice. She has been an advisor to many athletes and teams in different sports, working at all levels, from school and club to elite. As a competitive tennis player she knows the difference that nutrition can make to a performance.

Nutrition plays a key role in the optimal health and performance of all athletes. Many athletes have realised that unless they refuel their bodies with the right foods their training becomes difficult and their performance drops. Sports nutrition is not about magic pills, potions or special foods. It is about sound nutritional principles that help all athletes keep healthy, train hard, recover well and enjoy life. The British government's eight tips for eating well (October 2005) provide the nutritional basis that all athletes (and non-athletes) should follow. These guidelines are:

1 Base your meals on starchy foods
2 Eat lots of fruit and veg
3 Eat more fish
4 Cut down on saturated fat and sugar
5 Try to eat less salt – no more than 6g a day
6 Get active and try to be a healthy weight
7 Drink plenty of water
8 Don't skip breakfast

The role of nutrients during exercise

'Fuel' supply

Our muscles require energy to exercise and this energy comes from the food we eat. The two major fuel sources are carbohydrate and fat. Carbohydrate (CHO) is regarded as the 'premium' fuel as it is the only nutrient used when exercising anaerobically (without oxygen) or at a high intensity. Fats can only be used under aerobic conditions, so it becomes an important fuel source for endurance events, but less important for shorter events or high-intensity exercise.

Protein is only used as an energy source under 'extreme' conditions, such as when carbohydrate levels become low. Carbohydrate is the central fuel for the body. Once our body's stores of carbohydrate (muscle glycogen) are exhausted, our ability to use fat and protein is diminished and intensity has to decrease. Table 12.1 provides details of the amount of energy supplied by different fuel sources, while table 12.2 shows estimated energy expenditure for different sporting disciplines.

The ratio of fuels metabolised to provide energy depends on four main factors:

1 Intensity
The harder we train the more carbohydrate we use.

Table 12.1	Fuel provided by different nutrients
Nutrient	Energy supplied
1 g CHO	17 kJ
1 g protein	17 kJ
1 g fat	38 kJ
1 g alcohol (not an essential nutrient, but it does have an energy value)	25 kJ

2 Duration

This depends on the intensity at which we train and the amount of carbohydrate in the body. As our body's store of glycogen becomes low, protein is used more as an energy source. Branched-chain amino acids in the muscles can be broken down to glucose. Endurance athletes get approximately 10 per cent of their energy from protein whereas other athletes get only one to two per cent.

3 Diet

A high-carbohydrate diet helps restore glycogen storage and minimises lean tissue loss by decreasing protein usage. Dietary manipulation through carbohydrate loading can also increase glycogen storage. Higher glycogen stores enable an athlete to exercise for longer and sustain intensity levels.

4 Fitness level

Well-trained athletes have a better nutritional status. They have an increased ability to store glycogen, metabolise fats and sustain high-intensity exercise.

Therefore, the fuel supply is crucial to performance. Carbohydrate is the most important 'fuel' for athletes. Inadequate levels will compromise the training programme and, ultimately, the performance of all athletes (see fig. 12.1).

Table 12.2	Estimated energy expenditure in kilojoules (kJ)/minute					
Disipline		Body weight (kg)				
		50	60	70	80	90
Running	7 min/km	29	34	42	46	50
	5 min/km	46	55	63	71	76
	3.5 min/km	63	76	88	97	109
Cycling	15 kph	19	24	28	31	35
	25 kph	34	41	47	53	60
	30 kph	49	60	69	79	88
Swimming	Freestyle	32	39	46	52	59

Source: adapted from Melvin H. Williams, *Nutrition for fitness and sport*, William C. Brown Publishers, Iowa, 1988.
Note: to convert kJ to kCal divide by 4.2.

Figure 12.1 A high-carbohydrate diet maintains high muscle glycogen levels, while a low-carbohydrate diet depletes glycogen stores rapidly

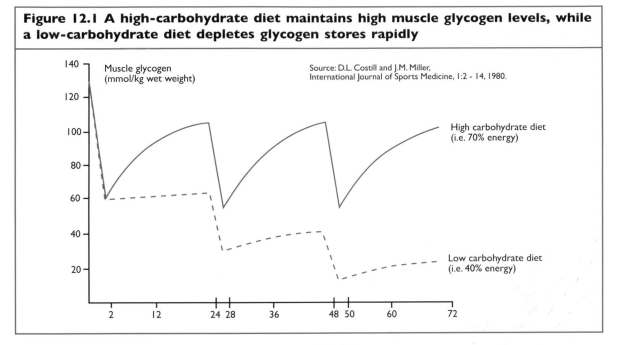

Vitamins and minerals

Vitamins and minerals are needed for the proper functioning of many body processes. If you choose your foods well, 5,000 kJ will provide all the nutrients you need. Many athletes have been led to believe that vitamin and mineral supplements will enhance sporting performance, yet scientific research has failed to substantiate this, except in cases where an athlete has an inadequate diet. Taking large amounts of some of these supplements has been shown to harm the health of athletes and impair their performance.

It is also important to put these nutrients into perspective next to our 'fuel supply'. For example, an 80 kg male triathlete training two hours daily requires:

1 Carbohydrate: 600–700 g = 38–44 oranges
   Vitamin C: 40 mg = 1 orange
2 Protein: 120–160 g = 550 g beef
   Iron: 10 mg = 350 g beef
3 Fat: 100–110 g = 3.2 l whole milk
   Calcium: 800 mg = 700 ml whole milk

Fluid

Water makes up approximately two-thirds of our body weight and is second only to oxygen in sustaining life. Without it we can only survive a few days. Dehydration has the biggest impact on the working capacity of muscles and temperature control of the body.

Dehydration occurs when fluid loss exceeds 1 per cent of body weight. Studies have shown that at 2 per cent body weight loss, VO_2max has decreased 10 per cent and endurance 22 per cent.

Failure to replace fluid during exercise can lead to heat stroke, heat coma and, eventually, death. The need for athletes to have an adequate fluid intake before, during and after exercise is critical to preventing dehydration and a decline in performance. Water is considered the nutrient most essential to athletes. *See* fig. 11.1, page 193, for the effects of fluid loss.

The training diet

The most important role nutrition has is to support the training and conditioning programme of athletes. A poor training diet leaves you feeling tired and lethargic, and unable to achieve desired or expected success. A good quality diet is essential to maximise your potential. No matter what success or level you have achieved as an athlete, if you know your diet is inadequate you could achieve more!

Nutritional considerations

Energy

Total energy needs are based on your weight, and the amount and intensity of exercise. The box below provides a relatively simple method of calculating energy needs.

Carbohydrate

The 'premium' fuel for the body and the limiting nutrient for endurance athletes. The athlete who fails to replenish glycogen stores on a daily basis will end up with chronic carbohydrate depletion and an inability to cope with training. The key to a successful training diet is ensuring adequate carbohydrate intake daily. Carbohydrate requirements are usually quoted as a percentage of energy. Endurance athletes should aim to get at least 55 per cent of their energy from carbohydrate, more if training for over two hours. The training diet should be made up of the following energy components:

CHO: 55–60%
Protein: 15–20%
Fat: 25–30%

For example, an active woman aged 35 and weighing 57 kg requires 15,500 kJ daily. If she trains for less than two hours daily, her carbohydrate requirement will be 55–60 per cent CHO. This will be 55–60 per cent of 15,500

Calculating energy needs

(a) Determine normal or ideal weight for you (kg).
(b) Multiply this by: 168 if adult and active;
                          252 if adolescent and active.
(c) Calculate total kJ cost of exercise (1 km swimming/2 km running/4 km biking = 525 kJ).
(d) Add (b) and (c) together to get an approximate level of energy needed to maintain body weight.

For example:
Woman, age 35, height 165 cm, 16% body fat
(a) Ideal weight = 57 kg
(b) Adult active = 57 × 168 = 9,576 kJ
(c) Weekly training schedule: 200 km cycling, 50 km running, 5 km swimming. Energy expenditure:

Cycling	26,250 kJ
Running	13,125 kJ
Swimming	2,625 kJ
Total:	42,000 kJ
Average per day:	6,000 kJ

(d) Energy needed daily = 9,576 + 6,000 = 15,500 kJ

kJ, or 8,525–9,300 kJ, which is 500–550 g CHO (1 g CHO = 17 kJ).

The major disadvantage of using percentages is that they are too vague and although athletes often know the percentages of carbohydrate to include, they are unable to convert that to the meals they actually prepare and eat. A more recent method of calculating carbohydrate requirements uses body weight and time spent exercising.

(a) Training less than 60 min: 5–6 g CHO per kg body weight per day
(b) Training 60–120 min: 7–8 g CHO per kg body weight per day
(c) Training more than 120 min: 9–10 g CHO per kg body weight per day

Table 12.3	Daily meal plan supplying 550 g carbohydrate (CHO)		
Meal/food	CHO (g)	Protein (g)	Fat (g)
Breakfast			
Before training			
200 ml weak fruit juice	10	–	–
200 g low-fat yoghurt	25	8	4
After training			
200 ml fruit juice	20	–	–
3 Weetabix, 250 ml skimmed milk	50	12	4
2 slices toast, margarine, jam	35	4	8
Lunch			
Filled roll (or 3 slices bread) and margarine	40	6	12
75 g salmon, salad	–	20	6
2 tsp salad dressing	2	3	3
1 large banana, 1 other fruit	35	–	–
Pre-training			
500 ml 5–10% CHO drink	35	–	–
Low-fat muesli bar	25	2	4
During training			
Minimum 500 ml CHO drink	35	–	–
Post-training			
200 ml 20% CHO drink	40	–	–
Large banana	25	–	–
Dinner			
Fruit juice, 200 ml	20	–	–
200 g pasta with sauce	75	12	12
100 g broccoli/cauliflower/tomato	5	–	–
100 g peas/corn/carrot	10	4	–
100 g lean beef	–	23	16
225 g fruit salad	25	–	–
125 ml custard	15	4	4
Supper			
Cup of Horlicks, skimmed milk	6	1	3
2 fruit biscuits	15	4	1
Milk in 4 cups tea and coffee	6	4	4
Totals (g)	**554**	**107**	**81**

Total energy (kj):
CHO: 554 × 17 = 9,418: 68% total energy
Protein: 104 × 17 = 1,768: 13% total energy
Fat: 71 × 38 = 2,698: 19% total energy
Total energy = 13,884

For example, a 57 kg woman training 2.5 hours per day requires 9–10 g CHO x 57 kg = 510–570 g CHO.

Work out a meal pattern to suit you, taking into account your training schedule and food habits. Spread your carbohydrate intake throughout the day, for example:

Breakfast and morning tea = 150 g
Lunch and afternoon tea = 200 g
Dinner = 150 g

Protein

Although it is not considered a good fuel source, endurance athletes use considerable amounts of protein due to the length of time spent exercising and the resulting low glycogen levels. Protein's prime function is to repair, build and maintain tissue and the more training an athlete does, or the higher the intensity they work at, the more tissue damage that is done. It is essential that athletes consume enough good quality protein to aid in their recovery from hard training. With much of the emphasis in meal plans on adequate carbohydrate intake, athletes can unintentionally have marginal protein intakes.

The protein requirement for endurance athletes has been established at 1.5–2.0 g per kg body weight per day. For example, a woman

Table 12.4	Common foods supplying 50 g of CHO (all measurements are approximate)
Breads and cereals	**Fruit and vegetables**
4 slices wholemeal bread 2 English muffins 1 1/3 medium bread rolls 6 rice cakes 20 water crackers 100 g cereal 60 g porridge oats 100 g muesli 1? muffins or scones	2 large bananas 3 other fruit 75 g dried fruit 9 dried apricots 2 medium potatoes 300 g corn
Pasta, grains and pulses	**Juices**
170 g pasta or rice 400 g baked beans 300 g kidney beans	600 ml fruit juice 500 ml soft drink 700 ml sports drink (5–10%) 200 ml sports drink (20–25%)
Snacks and confectionery	**Milk and dairy products**
7 plain biscuits 5 chocolate biscuits* 2 long or 4 small muesli bars* 150 g chocolate* 50 g sugar/boiled sweets 100 g potato crisps/corn chips 5 tbsp honey/jam	500 ml semi-skimmed milk 2 x 200 g low-fat yoghurt 400 ml custard* 225 g creamy rice* 225 g fruit dessert* 3? scoops (210 g) ice cream*

*Use lower fat options; if none, limit usage

weighing 57 kg requires 85–115 g of protein each day.

Protein needs can be achieved quite easily with a well-balanced diet (*see* table 12.5 for some good sources of protein). There is little need for protein supplement for most athletes.

Fat

Most athletes could lower the fat content of their diet (*see* table 12.6 for the fat content of common foods). There are several good reasons for doing this.

1 Fat often replaces carbohydrate. Fat contains twice as much energy as carbohydrate, leaves you feeling fuller for longer and depresses your desire to eat. This can be detrimental to an athlete with a high carbohydrate need. For example, 50 g of potato crisps has 25 g carbohydrate, 18 g fat. The fat content of the crisps is providing 62 per cent more energy than if you ate one large banana.

2 Fat is not good for your health. Many of the chronic age-related diseases (obesity, heart disease, some cancers) may be related to high-fat diets.

Vitamins and minerals

A diet that supplies enough energy, carbohydrate, protein and fat has plenty of variety and should meet all vitamin and mineral requirements. As already mentioned, in most cases the use of supplements is unwarranted. But if you decide to use supplements, use a multivitamin and mineral supplement in the dosages recommended.

Table 12.5 Protein sources	
Food	Protein (g)
1 small fillet steak (80g)	24
1 small chicken breast (80g)	19
4 slices of turkey breast (80g)	20
1 small salmon fillet (100g)	20
1 small tin of tuna (100g)	24
1 slice cheddar cheese (40g)	10
2 tablespoons cottage cheese (112g)	15
1 glass skimmed milk	7
1 carton yoghurt (150g)	6
1 egg	8
1 tablespoon peanut butter (20g)	10
3 tablespoons cooked lentils (120g)	9
1 Quorn burger (50g)	6
2 slices wholemeal bread	6
1 serving cooked pasta (230g)	7
1 scoop Casilan protein powder	14
1 protein sports bar	15*

* Values may vary depending on brand
Source: McCance and Widdowson's The Composition of Food (6th edition) Royal Society of Chemistry/Food Standards Agency (2002).

Table 12.6 Protein sources	
Food	Fat (g)
1 croissant	10
1 slice chocolate cake	21
1 packet crisps	10
1 tablespoon mayonnaise	23
1 knob butter	8
Quarter pounder with cheese	26
Cheese and tomato pizza (medium)	35
Confectionery bar	12
1 slice cheese (40g)	14
Small portion chips	9
1 flapjack	19
1 cereal bar	8

Source: McCance and Widdowson's The Composition of Food (6th edition) Royal Society of Chemistry/Food Standards Agency (2002).

Nutritional tips to lower fat intake

1 Keep high-fat foods to a minimum. Examples of high-fat foods include: most takeaway meals, pies, pastries, chocolate, potato crisps, many snack bars, cakes, biscuits, salad and oil dressings, luncheon sausage, salami, sausages, croissants, most desserts. If you can eliminate these foods from your diet most of the time, you will better manage your fat intake. It is important to read food labels. Use 3 g fat per 100 g or 30 kJ per 100 kJ as a guide as to what is satisfactory.

2 Replace high-fat foods with low-fat options. For example, replace whole milk with skimmed or semi-skimmed; replace cheddar cheese with Edam, mozzarella, reduced fat cheese, cottage cheese, quark, ricotta, fromage frais; replace ice cream with low-fat varieties of frozen yoghurt; replace butter and margarine with low-fat spread; make sure meats are lean or low-fat processed meats. Always be on the lookout for new products when shopping.

3 Use low-fat cooking methods. Grill, bake, steam or microwave when you can, and do not add unnecessary oil or butter (if you do have to use them, do so in minimal amounts).

4 Modify common recipes. For salad dressing, use plain low-fat yoghurt, or add a small amount of ordinary dressing and flavour with lemon juice and herbs. For mashed potato use skimmed or semi-skimmed milk and a small amount of low-fat spread. For white sauces use a low-fat spread, skimmed or semi-skimmed milk, and a small amount of cheese. For cream sauces for pasta use low-fat yoghurt or fromage frais. For meat dishes try decreasing the meat content by adding beans, pasta, rice, vegetables and sauces.

There are two minerals that are of concern to the athlete, for reasons of both performance and health: iron and calcium.

Iron

This mineral is an integral part of the oxygen supply system. It is found in the haemoglobin of red blood cells, which transport oxygen around the body. Low haemoglobin levels resulting from iron deficiency anaemia will seriously affect aerobic training. A blood test which measures serum ferritin (the body's iron store) should be done regularly (at least annually by athletes, especially endurance-trained athletes training two hours a day or more). For athletes who have been anaemic or who have marginal iron levels, checks should be done several times a year. At particular risk of low iron stores are women athletes, teenage athletes, endurance athletes, athletes with low energy intake and athletes not eating red meat.

Iron deficiency is fairly common among endurance athletes. It is, in fact, the most common mineral deficiency in the Western world. Athletes, especially menstruating females, are at more risk of iron loss through exercise than most of the population. Inadequate dietary intake and food choices can also reduce iron absorption and contribute to iron deficiency. When iron deficiency is first diagnosed, iron supplementation is required. But it must be remembered that diet is the key to achieving a satisfactory and sustainable iron status in the long term. See table 12.7 for more information on the iron content of common foods.

Calcium

The risks associated with calcium deficiency are more to do with long-term health problems than short-term performance. Studies have shown that low calcium intake increases the risk of osteoporosis (thinning of the bones) in later life, particularly in females. To help prevent

Table 12.7	Foods providing 3mg iron (1/5 female RDA, 1/3 male RDA)
Food	
2 tablespoons bran flakes (15g)	
Half a tin baked beans (240g)	
4 slices wholemeal bread	
12 prunes	
45g cashew nuts	
Medium portion broccoli (150g)	

Source: McCance and Widdowson's The Composition of Food (6th edition) Royal Society of Chemistry/Food Standards Agency (2002).

Nutritional tips for adequate iron intake

1 Eat a variety of lean red meat at least three to four times per week; approximately 150 g per serving.

2 Eat cereals with a high iron content, wholegrain breads, pasta and rice.

3 Include vitamin C-rich food at each meal to enhance absorption of non-haemoglobin stores, for example citrus fruit and juice, kiwifruit, strawberries, green peppers, tomatoes.

4 Keep tea to a minimum (two cups daily!) as the tannic acid in tea reduces iron absorption by 50 per cent. Try to drink it between meals rather than at meals.

5 Polyphenols in coffee inhibit iron absorption by about 20 per cent. The oxalic acid in silverbeet and spinach also reduces iron absorption.

See also 'Iron deficiency', page 205.

osteoporosis it is important to have a good calcium intake throughout life, but especially in the teenage years and early twenties. The importance of this as a health maintenance strategy for athletes and non-athletes alike cannot be emphasised enough.

Many athletes have reduced their consumption of dairy products under the mistaken assumption that these products will greatly increase their fat intake. Instead, they increase their risk of developing osteoporosis and stress fractures, despite the increased calcium absorption associated with weight-bearing exercise.

Some female athletes, because of training levels, low energy intake and low body fat content, also develop a condition known as 'amenorrhoea' (they stop normal menstrual functioning). This increases the risk of osteoporosis and negates the effects of increased calcium absorption through exercising.

Daily calcium requirements are: adults: 600 mg; teenage females: 800 mg; amenorrhoeic females: 1200–1600 mg. The richest sources of calcium are dairy products; plant-based sources are not as well absorbed. Where athletes are unable to eat dairy products, a calcium supplement is recommended, especially for amenorrhoeic female athletes.

Fluid

Fluid is of prime concern to athletes as dehydration will compromise training. A hydration plan must involve fluid before, during and after all training and racing.

Recommended training hydration plan

2 hours before exercise: 800 ml
Every 20 to 30 minutes during exercise: 150–200 ml
After exercise: minimum 800 ml

3 It should be high in carbohydrate, low in fibre and include plenty of fluid.

4 It should be low in protein and fat (these take too long to digest and could cause gastro-intestinal upsets).

5 Avoid gaseous or spicy foods that may cause indigestion.

6 Use 'liquid' foods (fruit smoothies and commercial energy drinks) if you suffer from pre-race nerves. These can be eaten within two hours of the race as they leave the stomach more quickly.

Examples of pre-race meals

Breakfast
- Diluted fruit juice
- Low-fibre cereal, low-fat milk
- White toast, honey
- Pancakes with golden syrup

Evening
- Fruit juice
- Pasta with low-fat sauce and vegetables
- Small serving chicken, fish, lean red meat
- Broccoli, cauliflower, mushrooms

Supper
- Low-fat milk drink
- English muffin or crumpet with honey

Other nutritional pre-race considerations

1 If you are not carbohydrate loading two days before the race, place special emphasis on carbohydrate and fluid intake. Consume limited alcohol, if at all.

2 The last big meal should be twelve to sixteen hours before the race.

3 Two hours before the start of the race, begin your pre-hydration regime – 800 ml of water, diluted fruit juice or low-carbohydrate drink.

4 Fifteen minutes before the start, drink another 300–500 ml of fluid – for races an hour or longer use only plain water. Immediately before the race you can have 200 ml of low-carbohydrate drink. Early in these races fat metabolism should be promoted. For races under an hour, 500 ml of low carbohydrate drink can be used with no side effects.

Race fuelling

The two crucial nutrients for racing are fluid and carbohydrate.

Fluid

During the race the primary need is for fluid. It is important to drink plenty *early* because once you are dehydrated it is too late. Never use thirst as a guideline for fluid need – by then you are already dehydrated.

Fluid should be supplied at minimum rate of 500 ml up to maximum 1600 ml per hour. The more hot and humid conditions are and the more you sweat, the greater the fluid needed to be consumed. The rate at which the stomach processes fluids (gastric emptying) depends on a number of factors, such as quantity, concentration and temperature of fluids. Some recommendations are:

- 150–200 ml of cold (4–10°C) fluid should be taken every 20–30 minutes of exercise.
- For races under an hour plain water is fine.
- For races over an hour take a 4–8 per cent carbohydrate drink with 460–720 mg sodium and 120–195 mg potassium per litre. Diluted fruit juice and soft drinks can be used (1 part drink: 2 parts water) although they are not as suitable as they contain no sodium to aid absorption.
- If the concentration is too high or too much is drunk, it can cause gastrointestinal upsets

and retard both the gastric emptying rate and carbohydrate absorption.

- For races over three hours you probably need to have a combination of fluid and solid food to provide variety.
- Check what carbohydrate drink is provided during the race. If it is not a drink you have used, start using it in training to familiarise yourself with it. If you are using a different carbohydrate drink during the event, you will need to organise yourself to have it placed at the aid stations.

What type of solid food should be eaten?

Foods high in carbohydrate and low in fat which are easy to chew and easy to digest are best. Remember to try out any dietary changes or new foods during training first.

At present there is some interesting research being done on the glycaemic index of carbohydrate foods and how this glycaemic index may help the athlete. The glycaemic index measures how much glucose levels rise in the blood after eating carbohydrates. High glycaemic foods have a value greater than 85. Moderate glycaemic foods rate from 60–85 and low glycaemic foods rate below 60.

Foods with a high glycaemic index cause blood sugar levels to rise quickly after eating, whereas those with a low glycaemic index provide a steady supply of glucose over several hours.

Initial results show that using low to moderate glycaemic foods before long workouts, and high glycaemic foods during long workouts and for recovery, could help optimise your training and race fuelling. The box below provides a list of foods belonging to the three categories.

High-, moderate- and low-glycaemic foods

High glycaemic foods
- Bread
- Rice
- Bananas
- Raisins
- Carrots, corn, potatoes
- Exceed sports drinks
- Gatorade sports drinks
- Honey, glucose

Moderate glycaemic foods
- Grapes
- Oranges
- Pasta
- Sweet plain biscuits
- Oatmeal, oatmeal biscuits
- Potato chips
- Ice cream

Low glycaemic foods
- Apples, peaches, plums
- Dates, figs
- Legumes
- Fructose
- Milk
- Yoghurt
- Cornflakes, muesli, Weetabix

How much carbohydrate should be eaten?

Approximately 60 g carbohydrate per hour or 1–1.5 g per kg body weight per hour has been established as sufficient to prevent glycogen depletion. For example: a 57 kg woman in endurance events needs 60–80 g CHO per hour. With 500 ml of low CHO drink supplying 35 g, a further 25–50 g would need to be eaten.

207

Nutrition tips

1 Consume drink and food early. Drinking and eating small amounts often decreases the chance of gastrointestinal upsets.
2 Do not eat or drink too much carbohydrate or you will retard the gastric emptying rate, delay carbohydrate metabolism and nullify the effect you are trying to achieve.
3 Try all foods and fluids in training according to race conditions.
4 Never try any new food or drink on race day.
5 Keep use of high-fat foods to a minimum as fat takes five hours to digest. They can cause indigestion, nausea and vomiting.

The refuelling diet

No matter how hard you train, if you do not eat properly you will train and compete with a less than adequate fuel supply. An important aspect of this is refuelling after a hard race or training. The most important nutritional considerations are the rehydration of fluids and the replenishment of glycogen stores. The sooner these are implemented after training and competition the more rapid the recovery.

Nutrition tips for refuelling

1 If you become dehydrated it may take 24 to 36 hours to become fully rehydrated. Drink fluids liberally. Do not include alcohol until rehydrated and keep coffee to a minimum. Rehydration has occurred when weight is normal and urine is 'pale and plenty'. (If you are taking a vitamin supplement the urine will be coloured.)
2 For maximum glycogen resynthesis carbohydrates are needed within the first hour after exercise. Delaying carbohydrate intake for more than two hours can mean glycogen recovery will take several days.
3 Glycogen resynthesis is greatest in the first two hours after exercise. A rate of 1–1.5 g per kg body weight per hour is recommended.
4 After the first two hours a rate of 50–100 g over two hours is sufficient, or 600 g carbohydrate over 24 hours. Recovery can then be made within 24 hours.
5 The type of carbohydrate may influence glycogen recovery. High glycaemic foods appear to result in faster glycogen resynthesis initially. Simple and complex carbohydrates in solid or liquid form can be used during the first 24 hours. From 24 to 48 hours complex carbohydrates provide better glycogen recovery.
6 Consume adequate amounts of electrolytes, especially sodium and potassium. Commercial sports recovery drinks contain added electrolytes.
7 Many endurance athletes need to train themselves to eat immediately after exercise as they often have no desire for food. Consuming an adequate carbohydrate drink is fine.
8 The refuelling diet must be part of your daily training – always include a drink and some solid food in your training bag for immediately after exercise.
9 Remember to include good quality protein in your next full meal. Protein is needed for tissue repair from training and, when you are exercising more than two hours, is needed to replace protein that has been used as energy.

The recovery diet and the training diet are regarded as the two most important aspects of an athlete's nutrition programme. Without instigating the correct dietary procedures for recovery an athlete can end up being glycogen depleted, with a resultant drop off in training, an inability to increase intensity or duration, and an increased risk of injury.

Nutrition alone will not guarantee your athletic success. By following the nutritional principles set out in this chapter, however, you can ensure that your performance is determined by skill and training, not eating habits.

PART **THREE**

SPECIFIC SAMPLE
PROGRAMMES

Introduction

In this new edition, I have included updated training programmes which are now tailored to your specific performance level. Whether you consider yourself to be a recreational, advanced or elite athlete, there is a training programme to suit your needs. Also, keep in mind the tips that follow, consult a coach if you feel it necessary, and, most importantly, enjoy!

Some people mistakenly think that the closer you follow a training programme, the better the chances of top performance. This is in fact not true. Listen to your body first, next look at the programme and then decide how you will train for the day or week.

It is useful to mentally divide your programme into three sections. In the first third you should be relaxed, then you should be diligent in the second part and focused in the third part. Don't fall into the trap of being overly focused during the early stages of your training. This will only make you feel exhausted and demoralised. Controlling your focus during the weeks of training will determine when you peak.

Cruise on your easy days so you can save up your energy for your harder (long, hills, speed) days. In the base phase of the training programme your long days have highest priority, with hills being next. If your aim is to improve your speed in long distance events, the 'long' aspect of the training is still most important; this is followed by 'speed', then 'hills' and finally 'easy'. When focusing on speed phases for shorter distance events, 'speed' should be the highest priority, with 'hills' next and finally 'long'. Always think in your workouts, 'Am I going to be fresh enough for my next key session?'. You may even cut your workout short on an easy day to ensure that you are ready for your high priority session. However, never try to catch up a missed workout. If it's gone, it's gone. You will destroy the balance of your programme if you try to catch up on the training time that you have missed.

Keeping a log book

Log books are a useful tool as they ensure that you have a record of your training. If your training was optimal, you have evidence of how it was. You can then use your log book with some refinements for your next build up. This way you are learning which forms of training work for you and which are ineffective which allows far greater improvements in training from one build up to the next. Also, if you are having problems maximising your performance, a log book will act as a guide to discovering what your training errors are and help you to address them. However, do not try to keep your logbook numbers straight. Keep in mind that your programme is a plan, but the reality of training is always different. It is perfectly acceptable to miss around ten per cent of the programme.

Don't stick to your heart rates like glue. They are designed to give you an idea of average intensity. Try to spend most of your training time at the recommended heart rates, but you are not expected to maintain them all the time. There is nothing wrong with your heart rate going up because you went up a hill or you raced someone for 5 – 15 minutes. Remember also that recovery is very important. Without recovery there is no improvement and without improvement there are no increases in performance. Recovery is very important.

Be patient: while this programme will help your performance, it generally takes two to three build-ups to get everything running really smoothly. Learn as much as you can about how to train. The 'whys, whens and whats'. If you understand how to train, you will get closer to optimal training.

How to use the training programmes

The following information is designed to help you get the most out of the training programmes in Part 3. If you follow these instructions you will get far more performance change out of your training programme. Each training programme consists of a graph, a table and explanatory notes that directly relate to each programme.

The graph

The graph at the top of your programme gives you a visual representation of training volumes.

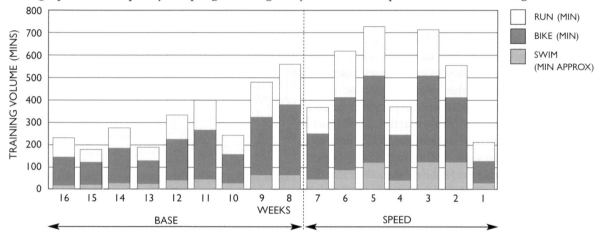

Legend:
- RUN (MIN)
- BIKE (MIN)
- SWIM (MIN APPROX)

The table

WEEK	10	9	8	7	6	5	4	3	2	1
SUBPHASE	1	2+3	2+3	2+3	2+3	2–4	2–4	2–4	2–4(5)	2–4(5)
MESOCYCLE		Build	Build	Build	Recover	Build	Recover	Build	Build	Recover
EFFORT		RELAX				DILIGENT		FOCUS		
TOTAL SWIM	20	60	70	80	60	90	44	120	80	34
TIME BIKE	90	260	380	480	130	580	120	460	300	50
(MINS) RUN	30	90	120	140	130	120	140	100	210	40
MON SWIM										
MON BIKE										
MON RUN										
TUES SWIM		1000E/T	1000E/T	1000E/T	1000E/T	1000E/T	1000E/T	1000E/T	1000RP/S	1000RP/S
TUES BIKE										
TUES RUN		40RH	60H	80H	100H	60RH	120H	40F	150F	30F
WED SWIM										
WED BIKE		60H/LC	80H/LC	100H/LC	60RH	120H/LC	60RH	120FBG	80FBG	
WED RUN		10E	10E	10E	10E	10E	10E	10E	10E	
THURS SWIM										500E/S
THURS BIKE		40H	40H	40H	40RH	40H	40RH	40RH	40RH	30E
THURS RUN		30E	40RH	40RH	20E	60RH	20E	60F	20F	20E
FRI SWIM		1000E/T	1500E/T	1500E/T	1000E/S	1500E/S	1000E/S	2000E/S	1000E/S	200E/S
FRI BIKE										20E
FRI RUN										10E
SAT SWIM	1000E/S	1000E/S	1000E/S	1500E/S	1000E/S	2000E/S	200E/S	3000E/S	2000RP/S	
SAT BIKE		40E	80FBG	100FBG	30E	120FBG	20E	120RH	60RH	HALF
SAT RUN	30E	30E	40H	40H	20E	40I1	10F	40F	40F	MAN
SUN SWIM										
SUN BIKE	90RH	120H/LC	180H/LC	240H/LC	TRI	300H/LC	120KM	180FBG	120FBG	
SUN RUN		10E	10E	10E		10E	15KM	10E	10E	

Subphase 3: high load

B   **BUNGY TRAINING**

Attach a bungy cord around the hull of your kayak. This creates a resistance. Develop more strength endurance. Try and keep your technique long and as much like your ideal racing stroke as possible.

Aim: Easy resistance training

SPEED:	LOW
STROKE RATE:	LOW
DIST/STROKE:	HIGH
SUBJECTIVE PACE:	EASY AEROBIC EFFORT HARD MUSCULAR EFFORT
HEART RATE:	NOT APPLICABLE

Subphase 4: load/speed

A   **ACCELERATIONS**

Move up to race pace, hold till you start to puff, then back off and cruise to recover details, as for AT.

Aim: Simulate race pace

SPEED:	MOVE GRADUALLY UP TO RACE PACE
STROKE RATE:	HIGH
DIST/STROKE:	HIGH
SUBJECTIVE PACE:	RACE PACE EFFORT
HEART RATE:	UP TO ANAEROBIC THRESHOLD AND THEN STOP

Subphase 5: low speed

UT   **UP TEMPO**

You should feel fast, strong, comfortable and in control. You should not be struggling. This is an effort at 3hr max race pace. Most people overdo this type of training. It should only be slightly faster than cruising pace.

Aim: Preparation for speed

SPEED:	MED
STROKE RATE:	MED
DIST/STROKE:	HIGH
SUBJECTIVE PACE:	EASY AEROBIC EFFORT HARD MUSCULAR EFFORT
HEART RATE:	UP TEMPO

Subphase 6: high speed

AT   **ANAEROBIC THRESHOLD**

This is max steady state pace or 20 min to 1 hr race pace. It should be hard but not unbearable! Most people overdo this type of training. You should be just below struggling.

Aim: Increase AT or RP

SPEED:	HIGH
STROKE RATE:	HIGH
DIST/STROKE:	HIGH
SUBJECTIVE PACE:	EASY AEROBIC EFFORT HARD MUSCULAR EFFORT
HEART RATE:	ANAEROBIC THRESHOLD

RP   **RACE PACE**

Note: This may also be part of subphase 5, depending on race duration. Race pace is defined as the effort level that you will use in the event. The aim is to simulate this effort level for short periods. Part of the goal of this type of training is to become accustomed to being able to reproduce the pace by feel so it is imperative that you reproduce the effort exactly and do not overdo it.

Aim: Simulate race pace

SPEED:	EXACT RACE PACE
STROKE RATE:	EXACT RACE PACE
DIST/STROKE:	EXACT RACE PACE
SUBJECTIVE PACE:	EXACT RACE PACE
HEART RATE AT LESS THAN 60 MIN:	ANAEROBIC THRESHOLD
HEART RATE AT MORE THAN 60 MIN:	UP TEMPO

Subphase 8: power

PO   **POWER ON (kayaks)**

Power on is basically rough water training. Many paddlers tend to become conservative in rough water and spend more time doing support and dip strokes. Power on training involves keeping power in the water irrespective of the rough water and balance. You may fall out a few times but you will get much better at rough water paddling long term.

Aim: Improve power in water irrespective of water conditions

SPEED:	MED
STROKE RATE:	MED
DIST/STROKE:	MED
SUBJECTIVE EFFORT:	MED
HEART RATE:	SHORT BURSTS AT UP TEMPO

ST   STARTS

Practice racing starts, including warm up prior to the race

Aim: Improve racing start ability

SPEED:	HIGH
STROKE RATE:	HIGH
DIST/STROKE:	HIGH
SUBJECTIVE EFFORT:	HIGH
HEART RATE:	NOT APPLICABLE

Tactics and extras

C   COURSE

Get used to the intricacies of the course that you will compete on.

Aim: Get used to open water swimming

SPEED:	EASY UNLESS OTHERWISE STATED
STROKE RATE:	MED
DIST/STROKE:	MED
SUBJECTIVE PACE:	EASY UNLESS OTHERWISE STATED
HEART RATE:	LONG SLOW DISTANCE UNLESS OTHERWISE STATED

W   WHITE WATER PRACTICE

White water training is to become accustomed to white water and reading water conditions.

Aim: Improve white water ability and reading

SPEED:	MED
STROKE RATE:	MED
DIST/STROKE:	MED
SUBJECTIVE EFFORT:	MED
HEART RATE:	LONG SLOW DISTANCE WITH BURSTS OF ANAEROBIC THRESHOLD

Note: White water may not always need to be on a river. You can use river mouths where there is a strong inflow/outflow; areas that you have identified as having the most fetch (the biggest waves); near a head-land; or between a large number of moored boats where there are waves and backslop.

Note: Big gear training should not be attempted by individuals under 16 years old. In this case, substitute with Hill training.

Cycling

Subphase 1: preparation

T   TECHNIQUE

Perform drills to improve technique

E   EASY

Aim: Improve technique and establish base fitness. Use coach or technique sheet as a guide.

SPEED:	EASY
CADENCE:	90–105 RPM
GEARS:	EASY
SUBJECTIVE EFFORT:	LOW
HEART RATE:	LONG SLOW DISTANCE

Subphase 2: load

RH   ROLLING CLIMBS

Rolling hills are climbs that are moderate or less than moderate in length.

Aim: Easy climbing

SPEED:	EASY
CADENCE:	50–70 rpm
GEARS:	EASY
SUBJECTIVE EFFORT:	LOW/MEDIUM
HEART RATE:	NOT APPLICABLE (APPROX LSD)

H   HILLS

Roll over hills in a small gear. Focus on the number and length of hills instead of technique.

Aim: Easy climbing

SPEED:	EASY
CADENCE:	50–70 rpm
GEARS:	EASY
SUBJECTIVE EFFORT:	LOW/MEDIUM
HEART RATE:	NOT APPLICABLE (APPROX LSD)

Hs   HILLS SPINNING

Climb long, moderate/steep hills in very small gear. Stay on top of the gear with very even pedal strokes. Maintain cadence and increase number, length and gradient of hills rather than changing into a harder gear.

Aim: Strength/technique

SPEED:	EASY
CADENCE:	65–80 rpm
GEARS:	VERY EASY
SUBJECTIVE EFFORT:	LOW/MEDIUM
HEART RATE:	NOT APPLICABLE (APPROX UT)

Subphase 3: high load

LC   LONG CLIMB

Climbing the longest hills you can find (longer the better)

Aim: Strength/technique	
SPEED:	EASY
CADENCE:	50–70 rpm
GEARS:	EASY
SUBJECTIVE EFFORT:	LOW/MEDIUM
HEART RATE:	NOT APPLICABLE (APPROX UT)

SC   STANDING CLIMBS

A standing climb is also like a long climb except you do the entire climb standing up.

Aim: Develop ability to stand for long periods

SPEED:	EASY
CADENCE:	50–70 rpm
GEARS:	EASY
SUBJECTIVE EFFORT:	LOW/MEDIUM
HEART RATE:	NOT APPLICABLE (APPROX UT)

HH   HUGE HILLS

As for hills only bigger. You need to be in the mountains to work on increasing the number of vertical metres ascended.

SPEED:	EASY
CADENCE:	50–70 rpm
GEARS:	EASY
SUBJECTIVE EFFORT:	LOW/MEDIUM
HEART RATE:	NOT APPLICABLE (APPROX LSD)

HBG   HILLS BIG GEAR

Climbing short hills of moderate gradient in a bigger gear than you would normally use. It should require a reasonable muscular effort. Travel 200–700m, 90% seated and 10% standing.

Aim: Strength endurance

SPEED:	EASY
CADENCE:	40–60 rpm ON HILLS
GEARS:	1–3 COGS HARDER THAN USUAL
SUBJECTIVE EFFORT:	MEDIUM/HARD
HEART RATE:	NOT APPLICABLE (APPROX UT)

Subphase 4: load/speed

FBG   FLAT BIG GEAR

Practice race position and maintain technique! Select a big gear (e.g. 53x16) but do not push too hard. It should not feel hard until you have been going for at least 20 min.

Aim: Build strength on the flat and teach the muscles to push a big gear

SPEED:	MEDIUM
CADENCE:	50–70 rpm
GEARS:	HARD

SUBJECTIVE EFFORT:	MEDIUM
HEART RATE:	NOT APPLICABLE (APPROX LSD)

TC   TEMPO CLIMBS

A tempo climb is the same as a long climb with tempo – imagine that you are training with a competitive friend to give you momentum!

Aim: Improve long climbing ability

SPEED:	EASY
CADENCE:	50–70 rpm
GEARS:	MEDIUM
SUBJECTIVE EFFORT:	MEDIUM/HARD
HEART RATE:	UP TEMPO

FUT   FLAT BIG GEAR UP TEMPO

This is the same as Flat big gear but now you have to increase the tempo.

Aim: Improve time-trial ability and strength on the flat

SPEED:	MEDIUM/HIGH
CADENCE:	70–80 rpm
GEARS:	MEDIUM/HARD
SUBJECTIVE EFFORT:	MEDIUM/HARD
HEART RATE:	UP TEMPO

BGTT   BIG GEAR TIME TRIAL

A big gear time trial involves riding at between 65 and 80 rpm in a bigger gear than you would normally use for a time trial. This is designed to improve your strength specifically for time trialling. Ideally, you start at a lower cadence for your first time trial and gradually move the cadence up as you get closer to your peak race.

Aim: Improve time-trial ability and strength on the flat

SPEED:	MEDIUM/HIGH
CADENCE:	65–80 rpm
GEARS:	HARD
SUBJECTIVE EFFORT:	MEDIUM/HARD
HEART RATE:	UT or AT AS STATED

A   ACCELERATION

Move up to an approximate race pace cadence and position with good technique. Reduce the effort when you start to puff. Accelerate or increase reps rather than holding race pace for longer or you will not get the benefit!

Aim: Power strength/acceleration

SPEED:	HIGH
CADENCE:	90–105 rpm
GEARS:	RACE PACE
SUBJECTIVE EFFORT:	HIGH
HEART RATE:	UP TO ANAEROBIC THRESHOLD

Subphase 5: low speed

UT   **UP TEMPO**

Practice race position and maintain technique! You should feel fast, strong, comfortable and in control. This is an effort at 3 hr max race pace. Most people overdo this type of training. It should only be slightly faster than cruising pace.

Aim: Preparation for speed

SPEED:	MEDIUM/HIGH
CADENCE:	95–105 rpm
GEARS:	MEDIUM/HARD
SUBJECTIVE EFFORT:	MEDIUM/HIGH
HEART RATE:	UP TEMPO

Subphase 6: high speed

AT   **ANAEROBIC THRESHOLD**

Practice race position, cadence and speed while maintaining technique! This is max steady state pace or 20 min to 1 hr race pace. It should be hard but not unbearable! Most people overdo this type of training. You should be just below 'struggling'.

Aim: Increase AT or RP

SPEED:	HIGH
CADENCE:	95–105 rpm
GEARS:	HARD
SUBJECTIVE EFFORT:	HIGH
HEART RATE:	ANAEROBIC THRESHOLD

RP   **RACE PACE**

Note: this can also be part of subphase 5, depending on race length. Race pace is defined as the effort level that you will use in the event. The aim is to simulate this effort level for short periods of time. Part of the goal of this type of training is to become accustomed to reproducing the pace by 'feel', so it is imperative that you reproduce the effort exactly and do not over do it.

Aim: simulate race pace

SPEED:	EXACT RACE PACE
CADENCE:	EXACT RACE PACE
GEAR:	EXACT RACE PACE
SUBJECTIVE PACE:	EXACT RACE PACE
HEART RATE FOR 20–60 MIN RACE:	ANAEROBIC THRESHOLD
HEART RATE MORE THAN 60 MINS:	UP TEMPO

Subphase 7: sprints

CR   **CRESTING**

Nearly full effort extended sprint, this should be like launching an attack on a hill, getting back on a bunch or taking a hill prime. Start 200–20 meters before the crest of the hill, followed by a 20 m attack up the hill and 20 m down the other side.

Aim: Improve ability to attack on a crest or go with an attack on a crest

SPEED:	HILL CREST ATTACK
CADENCE:	70–90 rpm
GEAR:	EXACT RACE PACE
SUBJECTIVE PACE:	EXACT RACE PACE
HEART RATE:	NOT APPLICABLE (SPRINT)

SPT   **SPRINTS (short sprints)**

Full effort sprint i.e. at the end of a road race, 100–300 m on the flat

Aim: Improve sprint speed

SPEED:	VERY HIGH
CADENCE:	90–120 rpm
GEARS:	HIGH
SUBJECTIVE EFFORT:	FULL EFFORT (HIGH)
HEART RATE:	NOT APPLICABLE (SPRINT)

Subphase 8: power

PWR   **POWER – Jump/Attack**

Nearly full effort extended sprint, attacking the bunch or bridging a gap. Don't get bogged down or buried by it, pull out before this happens.

Aim: Improve jumping ability

SPEED:	LOW TO HIGH
CADENCE:	LOW TO HIGH
GEAR:	HARD
SUBJECTIVE PACE:	FULL EFFORT (HIGH)
HEART RATE:	NOT APPLICABLE (SPRINT)

Subphase 9: overspeed

OS   **OVERSPEED**

Leg speed – little gear wind-out or sustained high cadence.

Downhill spinning sprint – accelerating down a hill in a small gear at a high cadence and trying to maintain a smooth pedal action by learning to contract and relax the muscles quickly. Try not to bounce on your seat. (50–200 m).

than race pace, getting the muscles fully ready for racing. Doing overspeed well above race pace is a waste of time. Do it at a speed just slightly above race pace.

Aim: Improve biomechanical leg speed and smooth pedal action

SPEED:	VERY HIGH
STRIDE RATE:	VERY HIGH
STRIDE LENGTH:	VERY LONG
SUBJECTIVE EFFORT:	LOW/MEDIUM
HEART RATE:	NOT APPLICABLE

Tactics and extras

C   COURSE

Get used to the intricacies of the course that you will compete on.

Aim: Get used to course

SPEED:	EASY UNLESS OTHERWISE STATED
STRIDE LENGTH:	LOW UNLESS OTHERWISE STATED
STRIDE LENGTH:	LOW UNLESS OTHERWISE STATED
SUBJECTIVE PACE:	EASY UNLESS OTHERWISE STATED
HEART RATE:	LSD UNLESS OTHERWISE STATED

P   PACING

Pacing is about setting up your strategic ability to get onto your race pace immediately and then hold it correctly through the race. Most people start too fast and come home too slow. Ideally, do a warm up beforehand to establish effort and rhythm. Then do the effort on an out and back course and try to get the same time for the outward part as the inward part – even splitting.

Aim: Ability to control pace

SPEED:	EASY UNLESS OTHERWISE STATED
STRIDE RATE:	MEDIUM UNLESS OTHERWISE STATED

STRIDE LENGTH:	LOW UNLESS OTHERWISE STATED
SUBJECTIVE EFFORT:	LOW/MEDIUM
HEART RATE:	LSD UNLESS OTHERWISE STATED

LD   LONG DESCENT

Climbing the longest hills you can find (the longer the better!)

Aim: get used to the impact of long descents

SPEED:	EASY
STRIDE RATE:	MED
STRIDE LENGTH:	MED
SUBJECTIVE EFFORT:	LOW/MED
HEART RATE:	LONG SLOW DISTANCE

F   DEAD FLAT

Run on dead flat terrain. It is important to train in all aspects of the race, even though flat running seems easy. This kind of running uses different muscles and these can get worn out if you do not train them. Normally, it is best to adapt to this aspect of training after building up hill running strength.

Aim: Adaption to flat terrain

SPEED:	EASY
STRIDE RACE:	MED
STRIDE LENGTH:	LOW/MED
SUBJECTIVE EFFORT:	LOW/MED
HEART RATE:	LONG SLOW DISTANCE

OR   OFF ROAD

Off road running is used to simulate the conditions that will be encountered in a race or may sometimes be used to reduce impact on the body. If you are doing an off road event in this programme please simulate the conditions as much as possible.

Aim: simulate off road terrain

SPEED:	LOW
STRIDE RATE:	MED
STRIDE LENGTH:	SHORT
SUBJECTIVE PACE:	EASY
HEART RATE:	LONG SLOW DISTANCE

Final words before you start

Points to note

1. Training should be evenly balanced to provide recovery time.
2. It is OK to miss 1–2 workouts in every 10 but try not to miss the important workouts.
3. Focus on recovery. Don't train if you are not recovered as it will only make you more tired and it could cause injury.
4. Make sure you do speed work, if you wish to do it, at the correct intensities. Doing speed work harder will not be beneficial. Training at the wrong intensity can actually have a negative effect.
5. Start out slowly and comfortably to avoid injury – overdoing training in the first four weeks is the main cause of injury.
6. Take what you think is easy and slow down by another 20–30 per cent just for the first four weeks. Don't try to be tough and don't race people! Your challenge is to train smartly.

Before you go out

Before I go training what part of the event am I training for today? What are my training, technical and tactical objectives today?

This is to ensure you train with clear objectives and purposes to ensure maximum return on time and effort.

After your warm up and during the workout

When I do this workout/while I'm doing this workout, am I the same or better than in a similar workout last week?

If your answer is the same or better, that's good, but if you think that your workout will be worse, reduce the intensity or volume of the workout. You can also decide to miss it in favour of your recovery. Training is about improving!

When you've finished your workout

What was good, what could I improve on, what will I need to do to get better next time?

This is to ensure that you learn and improve continuously.

This is how champion athletes operate. If you ask yourself the questions that champions ask themselves, you will tend to act like them, which in turn will raise your ability. There is your challenge!

Happy training!

TRIATHLON TRAINING PROGRAMMES

13

Triathlons are swimming/cycling/running events The distances for a standard triathlon are 1.5 km/40 km/10 km; for sprint distance, 750 m/20 km/5 km. The Ironman is an extreme endurance triathlon event, the first of which was held in Hawaii. This is still the most highly regarded but there are other Ironman Triathlon competitions no held all over the world.

The key things to remember are:

1. Judge your pace. Pace judgement is critical in the Ironman. In the 1988 Hawaii Ironman the racing heart rates of many athletes were monitored. It was found that the heart rates of the elite competitors fluctuated by 10 bpm or less for the entire journey. The heart rates of lesser athletes, however, fluctuated a great deal more. The key to optimal performance is to maintain a steady pace (and HR) throughout the race.
2. Know your fluid and energy requirements. Devise a schedule and stick to it. Poor drinking/eating practices can destroy six months of excellent training no matter how well prepared you are physically. This cannot be emphasised enough – fluid and food must be consumed at the right time. For instance, when you come out of the water you will be slightly dehydrated – swallowing sea water doesn't count! Rectify this as soon as you get on your bike.
3. Study the tide. Work out whether the tide is coming in or going out and if this will influence the best starting position for the swim. If you are in the wrong place you might get pushed off course by the tide and find you are swimming against it. This is extra work you don't need! Do your homework and use the tide to your advantage if possible.
4. Wind on the course. This has nothing to do with diet! In some events there is a tail wind for a significant stretch of the cycling section. Less experienced athletes often don't know this and they worry they have started too fast and consequently slow down. Then, when they turn around they are pushing back into the wind resulting in a less than optimal time. When you are running with the wind, sponge more often – there is less evaporation in these conditions and you tend to overheat more.
5. Urinating during competition. Why do you never see top triathletes urinating? Think about it!

Changes in triathlon

Drafting

Drafting is now used in the cycle stage of some triathlons, making swimming and running training more important. Learn how to draft in the swim; learn the skills and tactics of cycle racing in a bunch, and learn how to run like hell!

Multiple coaches

For multiple discipline sports such as triathlon, having more than one coach can be very useful (particularly if each is a specialist in one of the disciplines). One problem, though, is coordinating the input of each coach into a structured and balanced programme. Often, each coach will emphasise their sport too much. This can lead to overtraining.

Try to set up your coaching so that the training for each discipline is complementary in terms of phasing, volume and intensity each week. Ensure each coach has the same goal!

Sport-specific training used in triathlon

Type (intensity)	When initiated	Effect	Example	Race use
Power	—	—	—	—
Intensive sprints	—	—	—	—
Extensive sprints	—	—	—	—
Submaximal	Speed phase	Improves max steady state race pace	4–6 x 6–8 min 4–1 min rest between or 20–30 min TT	standard, sprint, Half-Iron
Up-tempo	Late base, early speed, speed	Transition from base to speedwork or long distance race pace – Ironman speedwork recovery rate	1–2 x 10–30 min rest 10–20 min between	standard, sprint, Half-Iron, Ironman
Long slow distance	Base/speed	Improves ability to do mileage, builds training and tolerance and improves recovery rate	continuous	all
Active recovery	Base/speed	Assists recovery (only if needed)	continuous	all

Proportions:
1 Base – 100% long slow distance and active recovery; some speedwork may be used.
2 Speed – approx. 85–90% long slow distance and active recovery; approx. 10–15% up-tempo and submaximal intensity.

RECREATIONAL SPRINT DISTANCE TRIATHLON (750 M/20 KM/5 KM)

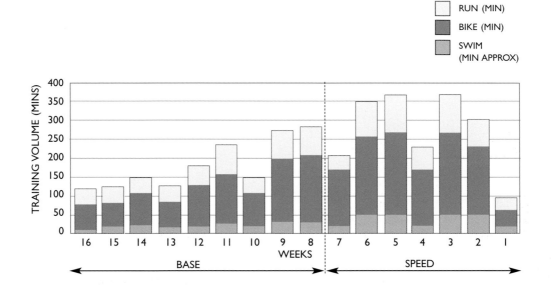

| RUN (MIN) |
| BIKE (MIN) |
| SWIM (MIN APPROX) |

WEEK		16	15	14	13	12	11	10	9	8	7	6	5	4	3	2	1
SUBPHASE		1	1	1	1	2	2	2	2+3	2+3	2+3	4+5	4+5	4+5	5+6	5+6	5+6
MESOCYCLE		Build	Recover	Build	Recover	Build	Build	Recover	Build	Build	Recover	Build	Build	Recover	Build	Build	Recover
TOTAL	SWIM	10	15	20	15	20	30	20	30	30	20	50	50	20	50	50	20
TIME	BIKE	70	70	90	70	110	150	90	170	180	150	210	220	150	220	180	45
(MINS)	RUN	40	40	40	40	50	55	40	75	75	40	90	100	60	100	75	30
MON	SWIM / BIKE / RUN							DAY	OFF								
TUES	SWIM																
	BIKE																
	RUN	20E+T	20E+T	20E+T	20E+T	30H	30H	20E	30H	30H	20E	40H+He	40H+He	30E	40H+He	30H+He	20E
WED	SWIM	200E+T	400E+T	500PB+T	400E+T	500PB+T	750S+T	500E+T	750PB	750RP	500E	1500RP	1500RP	500E	1500RP	1500RP	500E
	BIKE																
	RUN																
THURS	SWIM																
↓	BIKE	30E+T	30E+T	30H+T	30E+T	40H+T	50H+T	30E+T	60H	60H	60E	60RP	60RP	60E	60RP	60RP	30E
	RUN								10A	10A		10A	10A		10A	10A	
FRI	SWIM / BIKE / RUN							DAY	OFF								
SAT	SWIM	300E	300E	500E	300E	500PB	750PB	500E	750Co	750Co	500E	1000Co	1000C	500E	1000C	1000Co	500E+C
↓	BIKE						20E		20A	30A		30A	40C		40C	30A	15E+C
	RUN	20E	20E	20H	20E	20H	20H	20E	30H+He	30H+He	20E	30RP	40RP+C	30E	40RP+C	30RP	10E+C
SUN	SWIM																TRI
↓	BIKE	40E	40E	60E	40E	70E	80H	60E	90H	90H	90E	120H	120H	90E	120H	90E	RACE
	RUN						5E		5E	5E		10E	10E		10E	5E	EVENT

NOTES :

Suggested Practice Events: Baby Triathlon at the end of weeks 10, 7 and 4.

KEY

	REPS	HR
BIKE		
E = EASY		LSD
T = TECHNIQUE		LSD
H = HILLS		
HBG = HILLS BIG GEAR	1 – 3 X 500M	
FBG = FLAT BIG GEAR	1 – 4 X 10 MIN	
RP = RACE PACE	1 – 2 X 5 MIN	AT
A = ACCELERATIONS	1 – 10 X 30S	UP TO AT
C = COURSE OR SIMILAR CONDITIONS		
SWIM		
E = EASY		LSD
T = TECHNIQUE		LSD
PB = PULL BUOY	1 – 6 X 200M	LSD
RP = RACE PACE	1 – 5 X 200M	AT
CO = CONTINUOUS		LSD/UT
A = ACCELERATIONS		UP TO AT
S = SEA/LAKE SWIM		
C = COURSE OR SIMILAR CONDITIONS		LSD
RUN		
E = EASY		LSD
T = TECHNIQUE		LSD
H = HILLS		
HE = HILLS EFFORTS	1 – 6 X 200M	
RP = RACE PACE	1 – 3 X 4 MIN	AT
A = ACCELERATIONS	1 – 10 X 30S	UP TO AT
C = COURSE OR SIMILAR CONDITIONS		LSD

RECREATIONAL STANDARD DISTANCE TRIATHLON (1.5 KM/40 KM/10 KM)

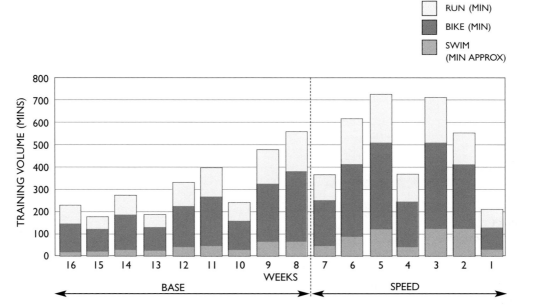

Legend:
- RUN (MIN)
- BIKE (MIN)
- SWIM (MIN APPROX)

		16	15	14	13	12	11	10	9	8	7	6	5	4	3	2	1
WEEK		16	15	14	13	12	11	10	9	8	7	6	5	4	3	2	1
SUBPHASE		1	1	1	1	2	2	2	2+3	2+3	2+3	4+5	4+5	4+5	5+6	5+6	5+6
MESOCYCLE		Build	Recover	Build	Recover	Build	Build	Recover	Build	Build	Recover	Build	Build	Recover	Build	Build	Recover
TOTAL	SWIM	16	20	25	20	35	45	25	60	75	40	90	120	35	120	120	25
TIME	BIKE	130	100	160	110	190	220	130	265	310	210	325	390	210	390	295	105
(MINS)	RUN	80	60	90	60	110	130	90	160	180	120	210	220	130	205	145	75
MON	SWIM	500T	500T	750T	500T	1000T	1000T	500T	1500PB	1500PB	1000T	2000PB	2000PB	1000T	2000PB	2000PB	500E
	BIKE																
	RUN	30E	20E	30E	20E	40H	40H	30E	50H	50H	40E	60H+He	60H+He	40E	60H+He	40H+He	30E
TUES	SWIM																
	BIKE	40E+T	30E+T	50H+T	40E+T	60H	60H	40E	75H+Hbg	75H+Hbg	60E	90RP	90RP	60E	90RP	75RP	60E
	RUN																
WED	SWIM	200E	400E	500PB	400E	500PB	750RP	500E	750PB	750RP	500E	1000RP	1000RP	500E	1000RP	1000RP	500E
	BIKE																
	RUN	20E+T	20E+T	30E+T	20E+T	40H	50H	40E	60H	75H	60E	90H	90F	60E	75H	60F	30E
THURS	SWIM																
↓	BIKE	30E+T	30E+T	30E+T	30E+T	40E	50E	30E	60E	75H	60E	75H+Hbg	90H+Hbg	60E	90H+Hbg	60H+Hbg	30E
	RUN	10E		10E		10E	15A		15A	20A		20A	20A		20A	10A	5E
FRI	SWIM								D A Y		O F F						
	BIKE																
	RUN																
SAT	SWIM	300E	300E	500E	300E	500PB	750PB	500E	750Co	1000Co	750E	1000Co	1500C	500E	1500C	1500Co	500E+C
↓	BIKE	20E		20E		20E	30E		30A	40A		40A	60C		60C	40A	15E+C
	RUN	20E	20E	20H	20E	20H	20E	20E	30H+He	30H+He	20E	30RP	40RP+C	30E	40RP+C	30RP	10E+C
SUN	SWIM																TRI
↓	BIKE	40E	40E	60E	40E	70E	80E	60E	100Fbg	120Fbg	90E	120Fbg	150Fbg	90E	150Fbg	120E	RACE
	RUN					5E			5E	5E		10E	10E		10E	5E	EVENT

NOTES :

Suggested Practice Events: Sprint Triathlon at the end of weeks 10, 7 and 4.

KEY

	REPS	HR
BIKE		
E = EASY		LSD
T = TECHNIQUE		LSD
H = HILLS		
HBG = HILLS BIG GEAR	1 – 3 X 500M	
FBG = FLAT BIG GEAR	1 – 4 X 10 MIN	
RP = RACE PACE	1 – 2 X 5 MIN	AT
A = ACCELERATIONS	1 – 10 X 30S	UP TO AT
C = COURSE OR SIMILAR CONDITIONS		
SWIM		
E = EASY		LSD
T = TECHNIQUE		LSD
PB = PULL BUOY	1 – 6 X 200M	LSD
RP = RACE PACE	1 – 5 X 200M	AT
CO = CONTINUOUS		LSD
A = ACCELERATIONS	4 – 10 X 30S	UP TO AT
C = COURSE OR SIMILAR CONDITIONS		LSD
RUN		
E = EASY		LSD
T = TECHNIQUE		LSD
H = HILLS		
HE = HILLS EFFORTS	1 – 6 X 200M	
RP = RACE PACE	1 – 3 X 4 MIN	AT
A = ACCELERATIONS	1 – 10 X 30S	UP TO AT
C = COURSE OR SIMILAR CONDITIONS		LSD

RECREATIONAL HALF-IRONMAN (PRE IRONMAN)

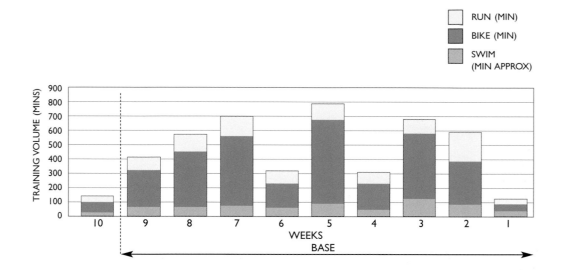

Legend:
- RUN (MIN)
- BIKE (MIN)
- SWIM (MIN APPROX)

WEEK		10	9	8	7	6	5	4	3	2	1
SUBPHASE		1	2+3	2+3	2+3	2+3	2–4	2–4	2–4	2–4(5)	2–4(5)
MESOCYCLE			Build	Build	Build	Recover	Build	Recover	Build	Build	Recover
EFFORT			RELAX			DILIGENT			FOCUS		
TOTAL	SWIM	20	60	70	80	60	90	44	120	80	34
TIME	BIKE	90	260	380	480	130	580	120	460	300	50
(MINS)	RUN	30	90	120	140	130	120	140	100	210	40
MON	SWIM										
	BIKE										
	RUN										
TUES	SWIM		1000E/T	1000E/T	1000E/T	1000E/T	1000E/T	1000E/T	1000E/T	1000RP/S	1000RP/S
	BIKE										
	RUN		40RH	60H	80H	100H	60RH	120H	40F	150F	30F
WED	SWIM										
↓	BIKE		60H/LC	80H/LC	100H/LC	60RH	120H/LC	60RH	120FBG	80FBG	
	RUN		10E	10E	10E	10E	10E	10E	10E		
THURS	SWIM										500E/S
↓	BIKE		40H	40H	40H	40RH	40H	40RH	40H	40H	30E
	RUN		30E	40RH	40RH	20E	60RH	20E	60F	20F	20E
FRI	SWIM		1000E/T	1500E/T	1500E/T	1000E/S	1500E/S	1000E/S	2000E/S	1000E/S	200E/S
	BIKE										20E
	RUN										10E
SAT	SWIM	1000E/S	1000E/S	1000E/S	1500E/S	1000E/S	2000E/S	200E/S	3000E/S	2000RP/S	
↓	BIKE		40E	80FBG	100FBG	30E	120FBG	20E	120RH	60RH	HALF
↓	RUN	30E	30E	40H	40H	20E	40H	10E	40F	40F	MAN
SUN	SWIM										
↓	BIKE	90RH	120H/LC	180H/LC	240H/LC	TRI	300H/LC	120KM	180FBG	120FBG	
↓	RUN		10E	10E	10E		10E	15KM	10E	10E	

NOTES :
Suggested Practice Events: Half-Ironman Simulation in week 4 Triathlon in week 6
Rest weeks: You should have a complete rest week before starting this programme

KEY

	REPS	HR
BIKE		
E = EASY		LSD
T = TECHNIQUE		LSD
H = HILLS		LSD
RH = ROLLING HILLS	I – 8 X I0 MIN	
FBG = FLAT BIG GEAR	I – 4 X I0 MIN	
FUT = FLAT BIG GEAR UP TEMPO	I – 3 X 500M	UT
RP = RACE PACE		AT/UT
A = ACCELERATIONS	I – 15 X 20S-1 MIN	UP TO UT
LC = LONG CLIMBS	I – 4 X I0 MIN	
C = COURSE OR SIMILAR CONDITIONS		LSD
SWIM		
E = EASY		LSD
T = TECHNIQUE		LSD
PB = PULL BUOY	I – 5 X 200M	LSD
RP = RACE PACE	2000M – 500H, 500E X 2	AT/UT
CO = CONTINUOUS		LSD
A = ACCELERATIONS		UP TO AT
LI = LONG INTERVALS	I – 4 X 500M	LSD
S = SEA/LAKE SWIM		
C = COURSE OR SIMILAR CONDITIONS		
RUN		
E = EASY		LSD
T = TECHNIQUE		LSD
H = HILLS		
HE = HILLS EFFORTS	I – 6 X 200M & I – 4 X 500M	
RH = ROLLING HILLS		
RP = RACE PACE		AT/UT
A = ACCELERATIONS	I – 15 X 20S-1MIN	UP TO AT
C = COURSE OR SIMILAR CONDITIONS		LSD

SEMI-COMPETITIVE HALF-IRONMAN (PRE IRONMAN)

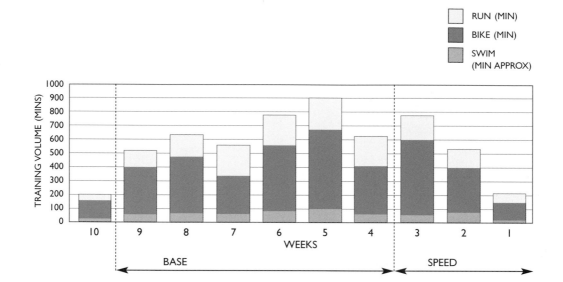

Week	10	9	8	7	6	5	4	3	2	1
SUBPHASE	1+2	1+2	2+3	2+3	2–4	2–4	2–4	4+5	4+5	4+5
MESOCYCLE	Build	Recover	Build	Recover	Build	Build	Recover	Build	Build	Recover
TOTAL TIME (MINS)	3	9	11	9	13	15	11	13	9	4
SWIM	20	60	70	64	90	100	64	60	80	24
BIKE	140	340	410	280	480	580	340	540	320	120
RUN	40	120	160	220	210	230	230	180	140	70
EFFORT			RELAX		DILIGENT			FOCUS		
MON SWIM										
MON BIKE		40RH	40FBG	40RH	40FBG	40FBG	40RH	40FUT	40FUT	40FUT
MON RUN		20RH	30RH	20RH	40RH/He	40RH/He	20RH	40RH/He	30RH/He	20E
TUES SWIM										
TUES BIKE		40RH	40H/LC	40RH	60H/LC	60RH/LC	40RH	60RH/LC	40RH/LC	30RH
TUES RUN		20E	20E	20E	20E	20E	20E	20E	20E	20E
WED SWIM		1000E/T	1000E/T	1000E/T	1000E/T	1000E/T	1000E/T	1000E/T	1000E/T	1000E/S
WED BIKE										30FUT
WED RUN		40H	60H	80H	100H	120H	60RH	120H	60RH	20E
THURS SWIM										
THURS BIKE		80RH	100RH/LC	60RH	100H/LC	120H/LC	60RH	120RH/LC	60RH	
THURS RUN		10E	10E	10E	10E	10E	10E	10E	10E	
FRI SWIM		1000E/T	1000E/T	1000E/T	2000E/LI	2000E/LI	1000E/LI	2000E/LI	1000E/S	200RP/S
FRI BIKE										20E
FRI RUN										10E
SAT SWIM	1000E/LI	1000E/LI	1500E/LI	200E/LI	1500E/S	2000RP/S	200E/S		2000RP/S	
SAT BIKE	60RH	60RH	80FBG	20RH	100FBG	120FBG	20RH	20E	60FUT	HALF
SAT RUN	30H	30H	40H	10E	40H	40H	10E		20E	IRON
SUN SWIM				1000E/T			1000E/T			
SUN BIKE	80RH	120RH	150H	120RH	180H/LC	240H/LC	180RH	300RH/LC	120RH	
SUN RUN	10E	10E	10E	90RH	10E	10E	120RH		10E	

NOTES :

Suggested Practice Events: Half-Ironman Simulation at the end of weeks 7 and 4

Long bike race at the end of week 3

Rest Weeks: You should have a complete rest week before starting this programme

KEY

	REPS	HR
BIKE		
E = EASY		LSD
T = TECHNIQUE		LSD
H = HILLS		
HBG = HILLS BIG GEAR		
FBG = FLAT BIG GEAR	1 – 9 X 10 MIN	
FUT = FLAT BIG GEAR UP TEMPO	1 – 6 X 10 MIN	UT
RP = RACE PACE		UT/AT
LC = LONG CLIMB	1 – 4 X 10 MIN	
A = ACCELERATIONS	1 – 15 X 20S-1MIN	UP TO AT
TT?? = TIME TRIAL FOR ??KM		UT
C = COURSE OR SIMILAR CONDITIONS		LSD
SWIM		
E = EASY		LSD
T = TECHNIQUE		LSD
PB = PULL BUOY	1 – 5 X 200M	LSD
RP = RACE PACE	2000M – 500H, 500E X 2	UT/AT
CO = CONTINUOUS		LSD
A = ACCELERATIONS		UP TO AT
LI = LONG INTERVALS	1 – 4 X 500M	LSD
C = COURSE OR SIMILAR CONDITIONS		LSD
RUN		
E = EASY		LSD
T = TECHNIQUE		LSD
H = HILLS		
HE = HILLS EFFORTS	1 – 6 X 200M & 1 – 4 X 500M	
RH = ROLLING HILLS		
RP = RACE PACE	1 – 3 X 4 MIN	UT
A = ACCELERATIONS	1 – 15 X 20S-1MIN	UP TO AT
C = COURSE OR SIMILAR CONDITIONS		LSD

PRE IRONMAN (BIKE EMPHASIS)

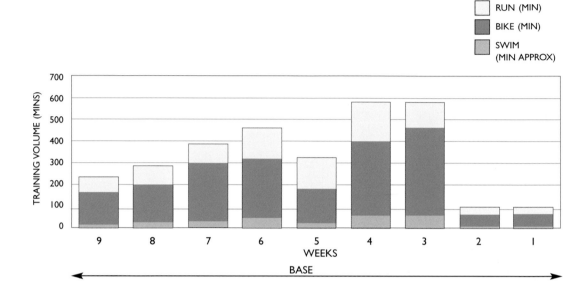

WEEK		9	8	7	6	5	4	3	2	1
SUBPHASE		1+2	1+2	2+3	2+3	2+3	2–4	2–4	2–4	2–4
MESOCYCLE		Build	Recover	Build	Build	Recover	Build	Build	Recover	Recover
EFFORT		RELAX		DILIGENT			FOCUS			
TOTAL	SWIM	18	28	36	50	28	60	60	8	8
TIME	BIKE	150	180	230	270	160	340	400	60	60
(MINS)	RUN	75	85	125	145	145	185	115	40	40
MON	SWIM	DAY OFF								
	BIKE									
	RUN									
TUES	SWIM									
↓	BIKE	30RH	30RH	40RH	40FBG	30RH	40FBG	40FBG	30FBG	30RH
	RUN	10E	10E	20RH	20RH	10E	20RH	20RH	10E	10E
WED	SWIM	400E/T	600E/T	800E/T	1000E/T	400E/T	1000E/T	1000E/T	400E/T	400E/T
	BIKE									
	RUN	30H	40RH	60H	80H	100RH	120H	60RH	30E	30E
THURS	SWIM									
↓	BIKE	30RH	30RH	40H	50H	40RH	60H/LC	60H/LC	30E	30E
	RUN	5E	5E	5E	5E	5E	5E	5E	5E	5E
FRI	SWIM	DAY OFF								
	BIKE									
	RUN									
SAT	SWIM	500E/LI	800E/LI	1000E/LI	1500E/LI	1000E/LI	2000E/LI	2000E/LI	2K	LONG
	BIKE								30K	BIKE
	RUN	30RH	30RH	40H	40H	30RH	40H	30H	15 - 20K	140 - 160K
SUN	SWIM									
↓	BIKE	90H	120H/LC	150H/LC	180RH/LC	90H	240RH/LC	300RH/LC		
	RUN	5E	5E	5E	5E	5E	5E	5E		

NOTES :

Suggested Practice Events: Ironman simulation in week 2

Course: The Ironman simulation should be carried out on the course or on 'like' terrain

KEY

	REPS	HR
BIKE		
E = EASY		LSD
T = TECHNIQUE		LSD
H = HILLS		
RH = ROLLING HILLS		
HBG = HILLS BIG GEAR	1 – 4 X 500M	
FBG = FLAT BIG GEAR	1 – 9 X 10 MIN	
RP = RACE PACE	1 – 3 X 5 MIN	UT
LC = LONG CLIMB	1 – 4 X 10 MIN	
A = ACCELERATIONS	1 – 10 X 30S	UP TO AT
C = COURSE OR SIMILAR CONDITIONS		
SWIM		
E = EASY		LSD
T = TECHNIQUE		LSD
PB = PULL BUOY		LSD
RP = RACE PACE		AT/UT
CO = CONTINUOUS		LSD
A = ACCELERATIONS		UP TO AT
LI = LONG INTERVALS	1 – 4 X 500M	LSD
C = COURSE OR SIMILAR CONDITIONS		LSD
RUN		
E = EASY		LSD
T = TECHNIQUE		LSD
H = HILLS		
HE = HILLS EFFORTS	1 – 6 X 200M	
RH = ROLLING HILLS		
RP = RACE PACE	1 – 3 X 5 MIN	UT
A = ACCELERATIONS	1 – 10 X 30S	UP TO AT
C = COURSE OR SIMILAR CONDITIONS		LSD

235

PRE IRONMAN (RUN EMPHASIS)

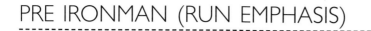

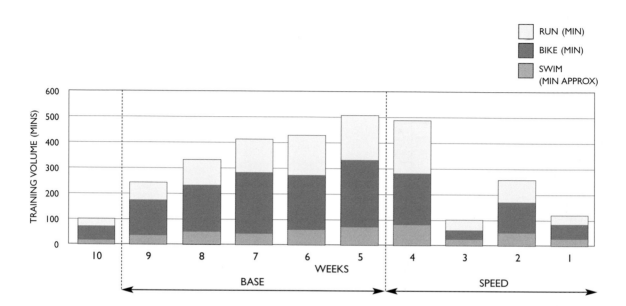

		10	9	8	7	6	5	4	3	2	1
WEEK		10	9	8	7	6	5	4	3	2	1
SUBPHASE		1	2+3	2+3	2+3	2–4	2–4	2–4(5)	2–4(5)	2–4(5)	2–4(5)
MESOCYCLE		Build	Build	Build	Recover	Build	Build	Build	Recover	Build	Recover
EFFORT		RELAX				DILIGENT		FOCUS			
TOTAL	SWIM	10	36	50	40	60	70	80	20	50	24
TIME	BIKE	60	140	180	240	210	260	200	40	120	60
(MINS)	RUN	30	72	104	132	155	180	210	40	90	35
MON	SWIM	DAY OFF									
	BIKE										
	RUN										
TUES ↓	SWIM					1500E/LI	2000E/LI	2000E/LI	1000E/T	500E/T	1000E/LI
	BIKE		30E	40E	60E						
	RUN		10E	10E	10E	40E	40RH	40RH	20E	40RH	20E
WED ↓	SWIM		1000E/T	1500E/T	1000E/T						
	BIKE					60RH	80FBG	80FBG	40FBG	40RH	40E
	RUN		20E	30E	40E	10E	10E	10E	10E	10E	10E
THURS ↓	SWIM										
	BIKE		30E	40E	60FBG						
	RUN		10E	10E	10E	60RH	60RH	40RH	30E	40RH	30E
FRI	SWIM	DAY OFF									
	BIKE										
	RUN										
SAT	SWIM	500E/T	800E/T	1000E/T	1000E/T	1500E/LI	1500E/LI	2000E/LI		2000E/LI	200E
	BIKE										20E
	RUN	30RH	40H	60H	80RH	100H	120H	150H	10E	30E	5E
SUN ↓	SWIM										2KM
	BIKE	60E	80E	100E	120E	150RH	180RH	120RH	30–40KM	80E	80KM
	RUN	2E	4E	2E	5E	10E	10E	10E	32–36KM	10E	20–25KM

NOTES :

Suggested Practice Events: Long run in week 3.

Course: The Long run event should be carried out on the course or on 'like' terrain

Rest Weeks: You should have one complete rest week before starting this training Programme

KEY

	REPS	HR
BIKE		
E = EASY		LSD
T = TECHNIQUE		LSD
H = HILLS		
RH = ROLLING HILLS		
HBG = HILLS BIG GEAR	1 – 4 X 500M	
FBG = FLAT BIG GEAR	1 – 9 X 10 MIN	
RP = RACE PACE	1 – 2 X 5 MIN	UT
LC = LONG CLIMB	1 – 4 X 10 MIN	
A = ACCELERATIONS	1 – 15 X 20S-1MIN	UP TO AT
C = COURSE OR SIMILAR CONDITIONS		
SWIM		
E = EASY		LSD
T = TECHNIQUE		LSD
PB = PULL BUOY	1 – 5 X 200M	LSD
RP = RACE PACE	500H, 500E X 2	AT/UT
CO = CONTINUOUS		LSD
A = ACCELERATIONS	1 – 10 X 30S	UP TO AT
LI = LONG INTERVALS	1 – 4 X 500M	LSD
C = COURSE OR SIMILAR CONDITIONS		LSD
RUN		
E = EASY		LSD
T = TECHNIQUE		LSD
H = HILLS		
HE = HILLS EFFORTS		
RH = ROLLING HILLS		
RP = RACE PACE	1 – 6 X 200M & 1 – 4 X 500M	UT
A = ACCELERATIONS	1 – 15 X 20S-1MIN	UP TO AT
C = COURSE OR SIMILAR CONDITIONS		LSD

237

HALF-IRONMAN/IRONMAN DOUBLE BUILD UP

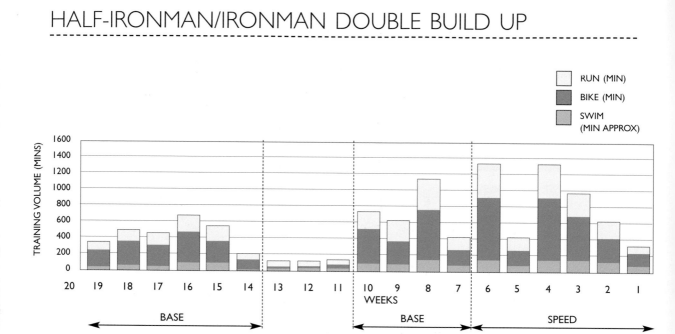

KEY:
- RUN (MIN)
- BIKE (MIN)
- SWIM (MIN APPROX)

TRAINING VOLUME (MINS)

WEEKS

BASE   BASE   SPEED

NOTES :

Suggested Practice Events: Half-Ironman Simulation in week 14
Triathlon or simulation in week 9, 7 and 5

Course: The Half-Ironman Simulation in week 5 and sunday training in week 2 should be carried out on the course or on 'like' terrain.

Rest Weeks: You should have a complete rest week before starting this programme

KEY		
	REPS	**HR**
BIKE		
E = EASY		LSD
T = TECHNIQUE		LSD
H = HILLS		
RH = ROLLING HILLS		
FBG = FLAT BIG GEAR	1 – 8 X 10 MIN	
FUT = FLAT BIG GEAR UP TEMPO	1 – 4 X 10 MIN	UT
LC = LONG CLIMB	1 -3 X 10 MIN	UP TO AT
A = ACCELERATIONS	1 – 15 X 20S – 1 MIN	
C = COURSE OR SIMILAR CONDITIONS		
SWIM		
E = EASY		LSD
T = TECHNIQUE		LSD
PB = PULL BUOY	1 – 5 X 200M	
RP = RACE PACE	2000M – 500H, 500E X 2	AT/UT
CO = CONTINUOUS		LSD
A = ACCELERATIONS	1 – 10 X 30S	UP TO AT
LI = LONG INTERVALS	1 – 4 X 500M	LSD
S = SEA/LAKE SWIM		LSD
C = COURSE OR SIMILAR CONDITIONS		
RUN		
E = EASY		LSD
T = TECHNIQUE		LSD
H = HILLS		
RH = ROLLING HILLS		LSD
F = FLAT		LSD
HE = HILLS EFFORTS	1 – 6 X 200M & 1 – 4 X 500M	
RP = RACE PACE	1 – 3 X 4 MIN	AT/UT
A = ACCELERATIONS	1 – 15 X 20S-1MIN	UP TO AT
UT = UP TEMPO	1 – 2 X 10 MIN	UT
C = COURSE OR SIMILAR CONDITIONS		LSD

Day / Discipline	1	2	3	4	5	6	7	8	9	10	11	12	13	14	15	16	17	18	19
WEEK	1	2	3	4	5	6	7	8	9	10	11	12	13	14	15	16	17	18	19
SUBPHASE	5+6	5+6	5+6	5+6	2-4	2-4	2-4	2-4	2-4	2-4				2-4	2-4	2-4	2+3	2+3	2+3
MESOCYCLE	Recover	Recover	Build	Build	Recover	Build	Recover	Build	Build	Build	Recover	Recover	Recover	Recover	Build	Build	Recover	Build	Build
EFFORT		FOCUS			DILIGENT				RELAX			REST			DILIGENT			RELAX	
TOTAL SWIM	74	120	140	140	64	140	64	130	84	80	20	20	20	24	80	80	40	60	40
TIME BIKE	160	300	560	780	200	780	200	650	300	440	60	40	40	120	280	400	270	300	210
(MINS) RUN	90	200	290	420	170	420	170	370	240	220	60	60	60	70	190	200	150	130	100
MON SWIM	2000RP/S	1000E/S	2000RP/S	2000RP/S	1000E/S	2000PB	1000E/T	2000PB	1500PB	1000PB									
MON BIKE	40E	40RH/A	40RH/A	60RH/A	80E	60RH	60E	80RH	40RH	40RH									
MON RUN	20E	30RH	30RH	80RH	30E	80RH	30E	60RH	40RH	30RH									
TUES SWIM																			
TUES BIKE	40RH	40FUT	80FUT	120FUT	60RH	120FBG	60RH	100FBG	80FBG	60FBG				40FUT	80FUT	80FUT	40FBG	60FBG	40FBG
TUES RUN	20A	30A	30H/He	40A	30RH	40H/He	30RH	40H/He	30H	30RH				20E	20E	20E	20E	20E	20E
TUES RUN				30RH		30RH		30RH	20E/T	20E									
WED SWIM	1000E	2000PB	2000PB	2000PB	1000E/T	2000PB	1000E/T	2000PB	1500E/T	1000E/T	1000E	1000E	1000E	500E	2000E/T	2000E/T	1000E/T	1500E/T	1000E/T
WED BIKE	30E	80F	120F	150F	80RH	150H	80RH	120H	100H	80H				30E	90H	80H	60RH	40H	30RH
WED RUN	20E													20E					
THURS SWIM	500A/S	1000RP/S	1000RP/S	1000RP/S	1000E/S	1000E/S	1000E/S	1000E/S	1000E/S	1000E/S									
THURS BIKE	30E	60FBG	120FBG	180RH/LC	60RH	180RH/LC	60RH	150RH/LC	120RH/LC	100RH					40RH	80H/LC	40RH	60H/LC	40H
THURS RUN	20E	20RH	20RH	20RH	20RH	20RH	20RH	20RH	20E	20E	20E	20E	20E		30E	30E	20E	20E	10E
THURS RUN			30RH	30RH		30RH		30RH	20E	20E									
FRI SWIM														500E					
FRI BIKE														30E					
FRI RUN														20E					
SAT SWIM	200A/S	2000E/S	2000E/S	2000E/S	200A/S	2000E/S	200A/S	1500E/S	200A/S	1000E/S	1000E	1000E	1000E	200E	2000E/LI	2000E/LI	1000E/LI	1500E/LI	1000E/LI
SAT BIKE	20E	40FUT	80FUT	120TT40	20E	120FBG	20E	100FBG	20E	80FBG				20E	40FUT	60FUT	40RH	60FBG	40FBG
SAT RUN	10E	30RH	30H/He	40H/He	10E	40H/He	10E	40H/He	10E	30H	30E	30E	30E	10E	40H	60H	40RH	40RH	30RH
SAT RUN			20RH	20RH		20RH		20RH		20RH									
SUN SWIM														2KM					
SUN BIKE	HALF	120TT40	180RH/LC	240RH/LC	TRI	240RH/LC	TRI	180RH/LC	TRI	120RH/LC				60KM	120RH/LC	150RH/LC	150RH	120RH/LC	90RH
SUN RUN	IRON	10E	10E	10E	OR	10E	OR	10E	OR	10E	40E	40E	40E	10KM	10E	10E	10E	10E	10E
SUN RUN					SIM		SIM		SIM		10E	10E	10E						

239

ADVANCED IRONMAN

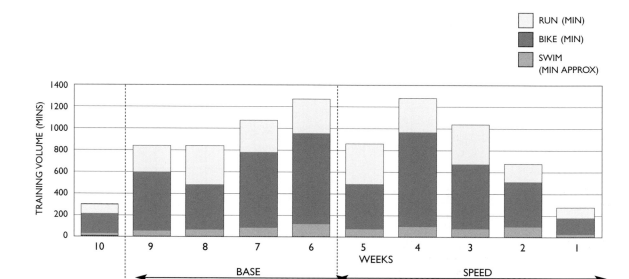

WEEK		10	9	8	7	6	5	4	3	2	1
SUBPHASE		1	2+3	2+3	2–4	2–4	2–4	5(6)	5(6)	5(6)	5(6)
MESOCYCLE		Build	Build	Recover	Build	Build	Recover	Build	Build	Recover	Recover
EFFORT		REST		RELAX			DILIGENT			FOCUS	
TOTAL	SWIM	30	60	70	90	120	80	136	80	100	34
TIME	BIKE	180	540	420	700	830	420	830	600	420	150
(MINS)	RUN	100	240	340	290	320	370	320	370	170	100
MON	SWIM										
	BIKE		40H	40H	60H	80RH	40RH	80RH	60RH	40RH	60RH
	RUN		40H	40H	40H/He	40H/He	40RH	40H/He	40H/He	40RH	30RH
TUES ↓	SWIM										
	BIKE		80FBG	60RH	100FBG	120FBG	60RH	120B/UT	120B/UT	80B/UT	60RH
	RUN		30RH	30E	30RH	30RH	30E	30F	30F	30F	30F
WED	SWIM	500E/T	1000E/T	1000E/T	1000E/T	1000E/T	1000E/S	1000E/S	3800E/S		1000RP/S
	BIKE										
	RUN	20E	100RH	120RH	150RH	180RH	120F	180F	120F	60F	30F
THURS ↓	SWIM										500E/S
	BIKE		100RH/LC	80RH	120RH/LC	150RH/LC	50RH	150RH/LC	120RH/LC	60RH	30E
	RUN		20RH	20E	20RH	20RH	20E	20RH	20RH	20RH	20E
FRI ↓	SWIM		1000E/S	1000E/S	1500E/S	2000E/S	1000E/S	2000RP/S	2000RP/S	2000RP/S	200A/S
	BIKE										20E
	RUN										10E
SAT ↓	SWIM	1000E/S	1000E/S	1500E/S	2000E/S	3000E/S	2000E/S	3800E/S	100E/S		
	BIKE		80FBG	60RH	120TT30	120FBG	60RH	120FBG	300RH/LC	180TT80	IRON
	RUN	80H	60H/He	60RH	60H/He	60H/He	60RH	60H/He	60RH	10E	MAN
SUN ↓	SWIM									2000E/S	
	BIKE	180RH/LC	240RH/LC	180FBG	300RH/LC	360RH/LC	180TT80	360TT80		60E	
	RUN		10E	90RH	10E	10E	120RH	10E	120RH	30E	

NOTES :

Course: All training in week 6, Sunday of week 5 and Saturday and Sunday of week 3 should be carried out on the course or on 'like' terrain

Race Pace: Ironman race pace, but no faster!

KEY

	REPS	HR
BIKE		
E = EASY		LSD
T = TECHNIQUE		LSD
H = HILLS		
RH = ROLLING HILLS		
HBG = HILLS BIG GEAR	1 – 4 X 500M	
FBG = FLAT BIG GEAR	1 – 9 X 10 MIN	
FUT = FLAT BIG GEAR UP TEMPO	1 – 6 X 10 MIN	UT
RP = RACE PACE	1 – 6 X 5 MIN	UT
LC = LONG CLIMB	1 – 4 X 10 MIN	
A = ACCELERATIONS	1 – 15 X 20S-1MIN	UP TO AT
UT = UP TEMPO	1 – 2 X 10 MIN	UT
C = COURSE OR SIMILAR CONDITIONS		LSD
SWIM		
E = EASY		LSD
T = TECHNIQUE		LSD
PB = PULL BUOY	1 – 5 X 200M	LSD
RP = RACE PACE	2000M – 500H, 500E X 2	UT
CO = CONTINUOUS		LSD
LI = LONG INTERVALS	1 – 4 X 500M	LSD
A = ACCELERATIONS	1 – 10 X 30S	UP TO AT
C = COURSE OR SIMILAR CONDITIONS		LSD
RUN		
E = EASY		LSD
T = TECHNIQUE		LSD
H = HILLS		
HE = HILLS EFFORTS	1 – 6 X 200M & 1 – 4 X 500M	
RH = ROLLING HILLS		
RP = RACE PACE	1 – 6 X 5 MIN	UT
A = ACCELERATIONS	1 – 15 X 20S-1MIN	UP TO AT
C = COURSE OR SIMILAR CONDITIONS		LSD

ELITE IRONMAN

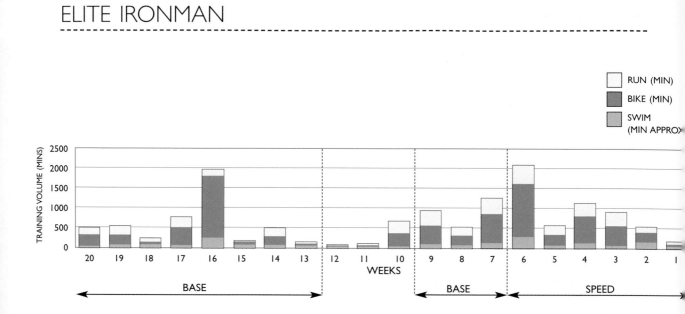

WEEK		20	19	18	17	16	15	14	13	12	11	10	9	8	7	6	5	4	3	2	1
MESOCYCLE		Build	Build	Recover	Build	Build	Recover	Build	Recover			Build	Build	Recover	Build	Build	Recover	Build	Build	Recover	Recover
TOTAL	SWIM	40	80	100	70	276	80	100	54	20	20	60	110	94	160	316	90	156	80	176	44
TIME	BIKE	300	250	40	450	1260	90	200	70	40	60	340	480	240	720	1290	280	670	510	250	80
(MINS)	RUN	160	260	130	260	440	40	220	40	50	60	290	370	220	390	480	230	320	360	150	80
EFFORT			RELAX			DILIGENT				REST				DILIGENT				FOCUS			
MON	SWIM	1000E/T	1500E/T	1000E/T	1500E/T	2000E/T	1000E/T	1000E/T	1000E/T			1000PB	1500PB	1000PB	2000PB	3000PB	1000PB	2000E/S	2000E/S	2000E/S	1000E/S
	BIKE	40RH			60FBG	120FBG									150RH			40RH/A	30RH/A		
	RUN	20E	20RH		30RH	40RH		30RH				40H	30H		30H	40H/He		30H/He	20H/He		30RH
TUES	SWIM			1500PB		2000PB	1800PB		1000E/S					1200E/S		2000E/S	1000RP/S			2000RP/S	500E/S
	BIKE	60FBG		40RH	60FBG	180H/Hs	40FBG		20E					60RH	120FBG	180FBG	40RH	80FUT	60FUT	40FUT	30E
	RUN	20RH	40RH	10E	20RH	40RH	10E	40RH	10E	20E	30E	40H	80H	10E	50RH	40RH	20E	30RH	20RH	20E	20E
	RUN		20E			20RH		20E				40RH	40RH		30RH	40RH					
WED	SWIM		1000E/S	1500E/S		2000E/S	1000A/S	2000RP/S	500A/S			1000PB	1000PB	1000PB	1000PB	3000PB	1000E/S			1000E/S	
	BIKE					60FBG	30E		30E						60RH					30E	
	RUN	80H	100H		150H	180H	20E	40RH	20E			80RH	100RH		150RH	180RH		180RH	120F	20F	
THURS	SWIM			1000PB		2000PB				1000E	1000E		1000E/S	1500E/S	2000E/S	2000RP/S	1500E/S	2000RP/S	1000RP/S	3800E/S	500E/S
	BIKE	40RH/LC	30RH/LC		50RH/LC	240H/Hs		40RH				120RH	180RH/LC		240RH/LC	240RH/LC		150RH	120RH		30E
	RUN	10E	20RH	120H	20RH	20RH		20E		30E	30E	20RH	40RH	120RH	40RH	40RH	90F	30RH	20RH	90RH/A	
FRI	SWIM					2000E/S	200E		200A/S							2000E/S					200A/S
	BIKE					120E	20E		20E							120RH					20E
	RUN					60E	10E		10E							60RH					10E
SAT	SWIM	1000E/S	1500E/S		2000E/S	3800E/S	2KM	2000E/S		1000E/S	2000E/S		3000E/S	3800E/S		3800E/S	1000E/S				
	BIKE	40FBG	40FBG		40FBG	180FBG	80KM	40FBG	HALF	40FBG	60TT30		60TT30	180FBG		40FBG	300RH	180TT80	IRON		
	RUN	20H	30H/He		30H/He	40H/He	30KM	40RH	IRON	40RH	40H		50H/He	40H/He		40H/He	60H/He	20E	MAN		
	RUN		20RH			30RH		20E	SIM	20RH	30RH		30RH	30RH							
SUN	SWIM																				
	BIKE	120RH	180H/Hs	TRI	240H/Hs	360H/Hs		120RH		40E	60E	180RH	240RH/LC	180RH	300RH/LC	360RH/LC	240TT80	360TT80			
	RUN	10E	10E		10E	10E		10E				10E	10E	90RH	10E	10E	120RH	10E	120RH		

NOTES :

Suggested Practice Events: Triathlon in week 18
Ironman Simulation in week 15
Half-Ironman Simulation in week 13

Course: All training in week 6 and on Saturday and Sunday of week 3 should be carried out on the course or on 'like' terrain

Work Days Off: It is advisable to take a day off from work on Thursday of weeks 9, 7, 3 and 4 and also on Tuesday of week 7.

Race Pace: Ironman race pace, but no faster!

KEY

	REPS	HR
BIKE		
E = EASY		LSD
T = TECHNIQUE		LSD
H = HILLS		
RH = ROLLING HILLS		
HBG = HILLS BIG GEAR	1 – 4 X 500M	
FBG = FLAT BIG GEAR	1 – 9 X 10 MIN	
FUT = FLAT BIG GEAR UP TEMPO	1 – 6 X 10 MIN	UT
RP = RACE PACE	1 – 6 X 5 MIN	UT
LC = LONG CLIMB	1 – 4 X 10 MIN	
A = ACCELERATIONS	1 – 15 X 20S-1MIN	UP TO AT
UT = UP TEMPO	1 – 2 X 10 MIN	UT
C = COURSE OR SIMILAR CONDITIONS		LSD
SWIM		
E = EASY		LSD
T = TECHNIQUE		LSD
PB = PULL BUOY	1 – 5 X 200M	LSD
RP = RACE PACE	2000M – 500H, 500E X 2	UT
CO = CONTINUOUS		LSD
LI = LONG INTERVALS	1 – 4 X 500M	LSD
A = ACCELERATIONS	1 – 10 X 30S	UP TO AT
C = COURSE OR SIMILAR CONDITIONS		LSD
RUN		
E = EASY		LSD
T = TECHNIQUE		LSD
H = HILLS		
HE = HILLS EFFORTS	1 – 6 X 200M & 1 – 4 X 500M	
RH = ROLLING HILLS		
RP = RACE PACE	1 – 6 X 5 MIN	UT
A = ACCELERATIONS	1 – 15 X 20S-1MIN	UP TO AT
C = COURSE OR SIMILAR CONDITIONS		LSD

TIME-EFFICIENT IRONMAN

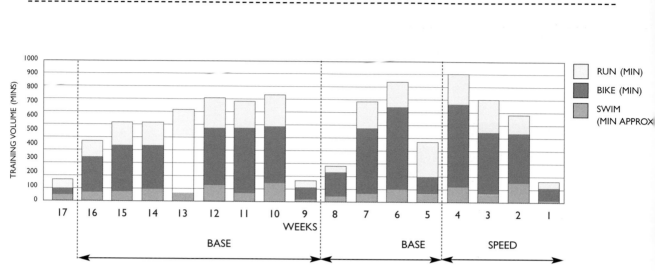

	17	16	15	14	13	12	11	10	9	8	7	6	5	4	3	2	1
WEEK	17	16	15	14	13	12	11	10	9	8	7	6	5	4	3	2	1
SUBPHASE		1+2	1+2	2+3	2+3	2+3	2–4	2–4	2–4	2–4	2–4	2–4	2–4	5(6)	5(6)	5(6)	5(6)
MESOCYCLE	Build	Build	Recover	Build	Build	Recover	Recover	Recover	Recover	Build	Build	Build	Recover	Build	Recover	Build	Build
EFFORT	RELAX					DILIGENT				REST	DILIGENT			FOCUS			
TOTAL SWIM	40	60	60	90	60	120	60	136	14	40	70	100	60	120	60	136	14
TIME BIKE	60	260	340	310	400	400	460	400	90	180	460	580	130	580	440	360	90
(MINS) RUN	60	110	160	170	200	220	200	220	50	40	190	180	240	210	230	130	50
MON SWIM		1000E/S		1500E/S		2000RP/S		2000RP/S			2000E/S			2000RP/S		2000RP/S	
MON BIKE																	
MON RUN																	
TUES SWIM																	
TUES BIKE		40FBG	40RH	60FBG	40FBG	60RH	40FBG	60RH	40RH		40FBG	60FBG	40RH	60FBG	40FBG	60FBG	40RH
TUES RUN			20RH		20RH		20RH		20E		20RH		20RH		20RH		20E
WED SWIM	1000E/S	1000E/T	2000E/T	1000E/T	2000PB	1000PB	2000PB	1000PB		1000E	2000E/S	1000E/S	2000RP/S	1000E/S	2000RP/S	1000RP/S	
WED BIKE																	
WED RUN	20E	60H	80R/H	100H	120H	150RH	120H	180H		20E	120H	150H	180H	180F	120F	90F	
THURS SWIM									500E/S								500E/S
THURS BIKE		60RH	60H	80H/LC	60H/LC	100H/LC	60RH	100R/H	30FBG		60RH/LC	000RH/LC	60RH	100RH/LC	40RH	60RH	30FBG
THURS RUN			20E		20E		20E		20E		20E		20E		20E		20E
FRI SWIM								200RP/S									200RP/S
FRI BIKE								20E									20E
FRI RUN								10E									10E
SAT SWIM	1000E/S	1000E/S	1000E/S	2000E/S	1000E/S	3000E/S	1000E/S	3800E/S	HALF	1000E/S	1500E/S	2000E/S	1000E/S	3000E/S	1000RP/S		
SAT BIKE		40H	60H	20E	60H	60FBG	60FBG	60FBG	IRON		60FBG	60FBG	30E	60FBG	60FBG	180TT80	IRON
SAT RUN	40E	20H	30H	10E	30H	30RH	30H	30H	MAN	20E	30H	30H	20E	30F	30F	10E	MAN
SUN SWIM																	
SUN BIKE	60E	120H	180H/LC	150H	240H/LC	180TT60	300H/LC	180F		180RH	300RH/LC	360RH/LC	80KM	360RH/LC	300RH/LC	60E	
SUN RUN		30RH	10E	60RH	10E	40RH	10E	10E					20KM		40RH	30E	

NOTES :

Suggested Practice Events: Half-Ironman in week 9

Course: Sunday training in weeks 5 and 3 should be carried out on the course or on 'like' terrain

Rest Weeks: You should have 3 complete rest weeks before starting this training programme

Race Pace: Ironman race pace, but no faster!

KEY

	REPS	HR
BIKE		
E = EASY		LSD
T = TECHNIQUE		LSD
H = HILLS	1 – 8 X 10 MIN	
RH = ROLLING HILLS		
HBG = HILLS BIG GEAR		
FBG = FLAT BIG GEAR	1 – 4 X 10 MIN	
RP = RACE PACE	1 – 3 X 5 MIN	UT
LC = LONG CLIMB	1 – 3 X 10 MIN	
A = ACCELERATIONS	1 – 15 X 20S-1MIN	UP TO AT
B = BUNCH RIDE	1 – 3 X 5 MIN	
C = COURSE OR SIMILAR CONDITIONS		LSD
TT?? = ??KM TIME TRIAL AT RP	1 X 80 KM	UT
SWIM		
E = EASY		LSD
T = TECHNIQUE		LSD
PB = PULL BUOY	1 – 5 X 200M	
RP = RACE PACE	2000M – 500H, 500E X 2	UT
CO = CONTINUOUS		LSD
A = ACCELERATIONS		UP TO AT
C = COURSE OR SIMILAR CONDITIONS		LSD
RUN		
E = EASY		LSD
T = TECHNIQUE		LSD
H = HILLS		
F = FLAT		LSD
HE = HILLS EFFORTS	1 – 6 X 200M & 1 -4 X 500M	
RP = RACE PACE	1 – 3 X 4 MIN	UT
A = ACCELERATIONS	1 – 15 X 20S-1MIN	UP TO AT
C = COURSE OR SIMILAR CONDITIONS		

DUATHLON TRAINING PROGRAMMES

14

Duathlons are running/cycling events usually comprising of a run, followed by a bike ride. In most situations this is followed again by another run. The distances are usually around 10 km/40 km/5 km or 5 km/20 km/3 km.

The key things to remember are:

1. Don't start too fast. It is always tempting to launch into a 'sprint start' but most people will find that they pay for this later in the event when fatigue kicks in. Try to pace yourself through the first run.
2. Stride Rate. Try to keep your stride rate constant throughout the run. Most people overstride going uphill and their stride rate drops. A loss of stride rate breaks your rhythm and makes your leg muscles tired. Imagine it like running up a flight of stairs two steps at a time!
3. Have a well-organised, practiced transition. The morning of the race, walk the transition area so you know exactly where you need to go.
4. Controlling the bike. Duathlons take either a time-trial or drafting format. In a time-trial format, make sure that you pace yourself and don't start to the bike section too fast. The adrenalin of the transition will still be surging through you! If you are in a drafting format duathlon, try not to do too much work at the front of your group and if you have to, try to 'soft pedal' for a brief time. Remain nearer the front of the bunch so there is less 'yo-yo effect' through the corners and on the hills, which will tire your legs. Make sure you are experienced at drafting in a group so that you save energy and try to anticipate the surging and braking. If you can smooth this out a bit it will save your legs still further.
5. Starting the last run. Most people run the first few kilometres too fast and 'explode' after that. Try to relax as you come into the transition area and start the run at a comfortable and consistent pace. Think about building on this pace after about 2 km.
6. Be aware of your hydration and nutrition strategies. This is particularly important in the longer events. The effect on how you feel and perform is significant.

Sport-specific training used for duathlons

Type (intensity)	When initiated	Effect	Example	Race use
Power	—	—	—	—
Intensive sprints	—	—	—	—
Extensive sprints	—	—	—	—
Submaximal	Speed phase steady state race pace	Improves max 4–1 min rest btwn or 20–30 min TT	4–6 x 6–8 min	Duathlon
Up-tempo	Late base, early speed,	Transition from base to speedwork	1–2 (10–30 min rest 10–20 min btwn	Duathlon long dist duathlon (4 hrs +)
Long slow distance	Base/speed	Improves ability to do mileage, builds training tolerance and improves recovery rate	Continuous	All
Active recovery	Base/speed	Assists recovery (only if needed)	Continuous	All

Proportions:
1 Base – 100% long slow distance and active recovery; some speedwork may be used.
2 Speed – approx. 85–90% long slow distance and active recovery; approx. 10–15% up-tempo and submaximal intensity.

SPRINT DISTANCE DUATHLON (5 KM/20 KM/3 KM)

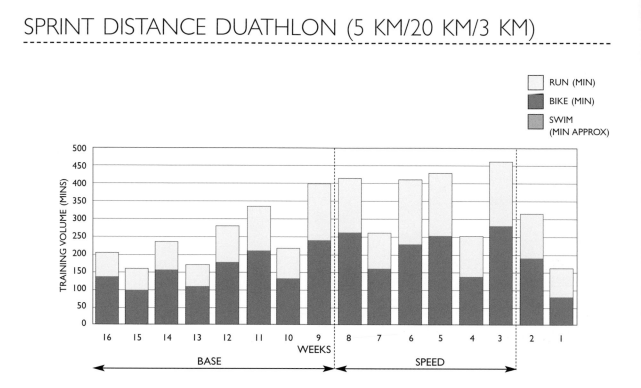

WEEK	16	15	14	13	12	11	10	9	8	7	6	5	4	3	2	1
SUBPHASE	1	1	1	1	2	2	2	2+3	2+3	2+3	4+5	4+5	4+5	5+6	5+6	5+6
MESOCYCLE	Build	Recover	Build	Recover	Build	Build	Recover	Build	Build	Recover	Build	Build	Recover	Build	Build	Recover
TOTAL TIME (MINS) BIKE	135	100	155	110	180	210	130	240	260	160	230	250	140	280	190	80
RUN	70	60	80	60	100	125	90	160	155	100	180	180	110	180	125	85
MON SWIM																
BIKE							DAY OFF									
RUN																
TUES BIKE	40E	30E	40H	40E	50H	50H	40E	60H+Hbg	60H+Hbg	40E	60RP	60RP	40E	60RP	40RP	30E
RUN																
WED BIKE																
RUN	20E+T	20E+T	30E+T	20E+T	40H	50H	40E	60H	60H	40E	60H	60F	40E	60H	40F	30E
THURS RUN					5E	10E		10A	10A		10A	10A		10A	10E	5E
BIKE	30E+T	30E+T	30E+T	30E+T	40E+T	50E+T	30E+T	60H	60H	60E	60H+Hbg	60H+Hbg	40E	60H+Hbg	40H+Hbg	30E
RUN	5E		5E		5E	10A		10A	10A		10A	10A		10A	10A	5E
FRI BIKE																
RUN							DAY OFF									
SAT RUN	10E		10E		10E	10E		20H+He	20H+He		20E	20C		20C	20E	10E+C
BIKE	20E		20E		20E	30E		30A	40A		40A	60C		60C	40A	15E+C
RUN	10E	20E	10H	20E	10H	10H	20E	10E	10E	20E	20RP	20RP+C	30E	20RP+C	10RP	10E+C
SUN BIKE	40E	40E	60E	40E	60E	70E	60E	80Fbg	90Fbg	60E	90Fbg	90Fbg	60E	90Fbg	60E	RACE
RUN					5E			5E	5E		10E	10E		10E	5E	EVENT

NOTES :

Suggested Practice Events: Baby Duathlon in weeks 10, 7 and 4

KEY	REPS	HR
BIKE		
E = EASY		LSD
T = TECHNIQUE		LSD
H = HILLS		
HBG = HILLS BIG GEAR	1– 3 X 500M	
FBG = FLAT BIG GEAR	1 – 4 X 10 MIN	
RP = RACE PACE	1 – 2 X 5 MIN	AT
A = ACCELERATIONS	1 – 10 X 30S	UP TO AT
C = COURSE OR SIMILAR CONDITIONS		LSD
RUN		
E = EASY		LSD
T = TECHNIQUE		LSD
H = HILLS		
HE = HILLS EFFORTS	1 – 6 X 200M	
RP = RACE PACE	1 – 3 X 4 MIN	AT
A = ACCELERATIONS	1 – 10 X 30S	UP TO AT
C = COURSE OR SIMILAR CONDITIONS		LSD

ADVANCED DUATHLON (10 KM/4 KM/5 KM)

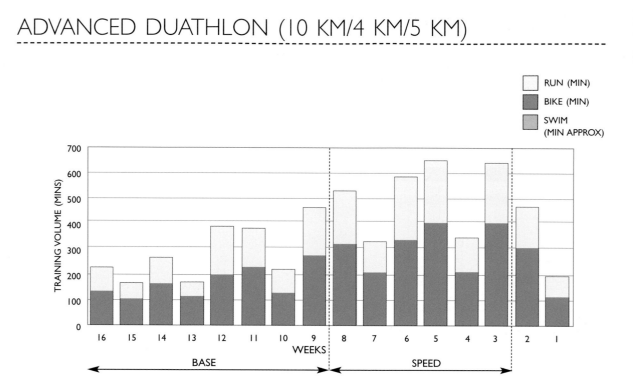

Legend:
- RUN (MIN)
- BIKE (MIN)
- SWIM (MIN APPROX)

WEEK		16	15	14	13	12	11	10	9	8	7	6	5	4	3	2	1
SUBPHASE		1	1	1	1	2	2	2	2+3	2+3	2+3	4+5	4+5	4+5	5+6	5+6	5+6
MESOCYCLE		Build	Recover	Build	Recover	Build	Build	Recover	Build	Build	Recover	Build	Build	Recover	Build	Build	Recover
TOTAL TIME (MINS)	BIKE	135	100	165	110	200	230	130	275	320	210	335	400	210	400	305	110
	RUN	90	60	100	60	130	150	90	190	210	120	250	250	130	235	165	85
MON	BIKE																
	RUN	30E	20E	30E	20E	40H	40H	30E	50H	50H	40E	60H+He	60H+He	40E	60H+He	40H+He	30E
TUES	BIKE	40E	30E	50H	40E	60H	60H	40E	75H+Hbg	75H+Hbg	60E	90RP	90RP	60E	90RP	75RP	60E
	RUN																
WED	BIKE																
	RUN	20E+T	20E+T	30E+T	20E+T	40H	50H	40E	60H	75H	60E	90H	90F	60E	75H	60F	30E
THURS	RUN	5E		5E		10E	10E		10A	10A		10A	10A		10A	10E	5E
↓	BIKE	30E+T	30E+T	30E+T	30E+T	40E+T	50H	30E	60H	75H	60E	75H+Hbg	90H+Hbg	60E	90H+Hbg	60H+Hbg	30E
	RUN	10E		10E		10E	15A		15A	20A		20A	20A		20A	10A	5E
FRI	SWIM	DAY OFF															
	BIKE																
	RUN																
SAT	RUN	20E		20E		20E	20E		30E	30E		40E	40C		40C	30E	10E+C
↓	BIKE	20E		20E		20E	30E		30A	40A		40A	60C		60C	40A	15E+C
	RUN	10E	20E	10H	20E	20H	20H	20E	30H+He	30H+He	20E	30RP	30RP+C	30E	30RP+C	20RP	10E+C
SUN	SWIM																
↓	BIKE	40E	40E	60E	40E	70E	80E	60E	100Fbg	120Fbg	90E	120Fbg	150Fbg	90E	150Fbg	120E	RACE
	RUN						5E		5E	5E		10E	10E		10E	5E	EVENT

NOTES :

Suggested Practice Events: Sprint Duathlon in weeks 10, 7 and 4

KEY	REPS	HR
BIKE		
E = EASY		LSD
T = TECHNIQUE		LSD
H = HILLS		
HBG = HILLS BIG GEAR	1 – 3 X 500M	
FBG = FLAT BIG GEAR	1 – 4 X 10 MIN	
RP = RACE PACE	1 – 2 X 5 MIN	AT
A = ACCELERATIONS	1 – 10 X 30S	UP TO AT
C = COURSE OR SIMILAR CONDITIONS		LSD
RUN		
E = EASY		LSD
T = TECHNIQUE		LSD
H = HILLS		
HE = HILLS EFFORTS	1 – 6 X 200M	
RP = RACE PACE	1 – 3 X 4 MIN	AT
A = ACCELERATIONS	1 – 10 X 30S	UP TO AT
C = COURSE OR SIMILAR CONDITIONS		LSD

MULTI-SPORT TRAINING PROGRAMMES

15

Adventure Racing usually involves multi-member teams navigating and route finding their way through multiple checkpoints in a variety of ways. These more commonly include mountain biking, kayaking, running/trekking and various rock climbing skills like abseiling. More unusual skills might include river rafting, coasteering, canyoning, mountain climbing and sailing to name a few. Most events are around 6 to 24 hours long but events can last up to 10 days. They have been made famous by iconic events such as Southern Traverse, Raid Gauloises and Ecochallenge. Expect to spend quite a bit of money on equipment and gear but the events are usually spectacular – expect amazing experiences!

The key things to remember are:

1. Always know where you are on the map. Map reading means you know where you are at all times and can predict what you will see next. Most adventure racers tend to read the map occasionally as they go along, moving as fast as they can, but you are far more likely to get lost this way.
2. Look after your feet. Most events take a long period of time to complete and the conditions play havoc with your feet – climbs and descents, trekking/running through mud and water. Make sure that your shoes are correct for the environment and that they have been well worn in. You should use quick-dry socks and read up on foot care before you go. The socks should be quick dry and used many times before and you know all there is to know about foot care. Foot problems are like a flat tyre on a car – not too serious for the car but it stops you going anywhere in a hurry!
3. Train with all your gear regularly. Carrying a pack and wearing all your gear is very different from going for a quick run or mountain bike. Make sure that you train with all your gear so you get used to it and understand how it affects you (e.g. a chafing pack strap)
4. Get used to long climbs and descents. These are an element of most adventure races and if you are not used to them they will cause your legs to 'blow up'.
5. Do not spend too much time at checkpoints and change-overs. This time passes by very easily so be strict and keep an eye on your watch!
6. Practice in all conditions. If you can, get used to the environmental conditions you think you will face. Also, do team simulations to practice working together and get all the logistics sorted out.

Sport-specific training used for multi-sport events

Type (intensity)	When initiated	Effect	Example	Race use
Power	—	—	—	—
Intensive sprints	—	—	—	—
Extensive sprints	Late speed phase	Improves extended sprint	4–6 × 1–3 rest to recovery bike race, initial run	???? bike ride initial run
Submaximal	Speed phase	Improves max steady state race pace	4–6 × 6–8 m 4–1 min rest btwn or 20–30 min TT.	All (small amount if in 4 hr+ races)
Up-tempo	Late base, early speed	Transition from base to speedwork	1–2 × 10–30 min rest 10–20 min btwn	All
Long slow distance	Base/speed	Improves ability to do mileage, builds training tolerance and improves recovery rate	Continuous	All
Active recovery	Base/speed	Assists recovery (only if needed)	Continuous	All

Proportions:
1 Base – 100% long slow distance and active recovery; some speedwork may be used.
2 Speed – approx. 85–90% long slow distance and active recovery; approx. 10–15% up-tempo and submaximal intensity

12-HOUR ADVENTURE RACE

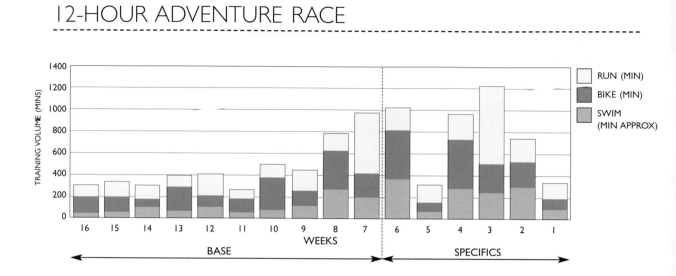

Chart legend: RUN (MIN), BIKE (MIN), SWIM (MIN APPROX). Y-axis: TRAINING VOLUME (MINS). X-axis: WEEKS 16 to 1. BASE (weeks 16–7), SPECIFICS (weeks 6–1).

	16	15	14	13	12	11	10	9	8	7	6	5	4	3	2	1
WEEK	16	15	14	13	12	11	10	9	8	7	6	5	4	3	2	1
SUBPHASE	1+2	1+2	1+2	2	2	2	2+3	2+3	2+3	2+3	2+3	2+3	4+5	4+5	4+5	4+5
MESOCYCLE	Build	Build	Recover	Build	Build	Recover	Build	Build	Recover	Build	Build	Recover	Build	Build	Recover	Recover
TOTAL TIME (MINS) — KAYAK	50	60	100	70	110	60	80	120	270	195	360	70	280	240	290	90
BIKE	150	140	80	230	100	130	295	140	350	215	450	80	450	270	240	100
TREK/RUN	100	140	120	100	200	80	130	190	170	570	220	160	240	720	210	150
MON KAYAK	20E+T	30E+T	40E+T	50B	60B	60E	60B	60B	60E	60B	60TP	60E	60TP	60TP	60TP	40E
MON BIKE																
MON RUN	20E+T	20E+T	30E+T	30H	30H	20E	30H	30H	20E	30H	40H	20E	40H	40H	40H	20E
TUES KAYAK																
TUES BIKE	40E+T	40E+T	50E+T	60H	40H	60E	60FBG	75FBG	60E	75FBGH	90FBGH	60E	60TP	90TP	60TP	60E
TUES TREK																
WED KAYAK	30E	30E	40E	40E	30E	30E	40E	50B	30E	60B	60B	40E	60B	60B	40B	30E
WED BIKE																
WED TREK	30E	40E	30E	40E	50H	30E	60H	60HH	30E	60HH	60HH	40E	90TP	60TP	60TP	30E
THURS KAYAK																
THURS BIKE	30E	40E	30E	50E	60E	40E	75H	90H	60E	90HH	120HH	90E	120H	120H	90H	60E
THURS TREK																
FRI KAYAK			ROPE			ROPE				ROPE		ROPE		ROPE	ROPE	
FRI BIKE / TREK						D A Y O F F										
SAT KAYAK	20E	30E	60E	30E	80E	30E	40E	100E	SIM	60E	120TP	20E	60E	120TP	20E	RACE
SAT BIKE	20E	30E		30E		30E	40E		SIM	60E		20E	60E		20E	RACE
SAT TREK	20E	30E		30E		30E	40E			60E		20E	60E		20E	
SUN KAYAK																
SUN BIKE	60E	30E		90E	SIM		120GNC	SIM	150ECN		SIM	180DEGC			60E	RACE
SUN TREK	60E	90E	60E			120NC			150NC	180ENGC				240DEGC	60E	

NOTES :

Suggested Practice Events: 12hr Adventure Race Simulation in weeks 11, 8 and 5

Rope: Practise all your rope work (e.g. abseiling) on this day.

Trekking: Assume for all trekking training that you use footwear, clothing and pack that will be used in the race.

KEY

	REPS	HR
BIKE		
E = EASY		LSD
T = TECHNIQUE		LSD
H = HILLS		
HH = REALLY BIG HILLS		
C = COURSE OR SIMILAR CONDITIONS		LSD
RP = RACE PACE	1 – 6 X 10 MIN	UT
KAYAK		
E = EASY		LSD
T = TECHNIQUE		LSD
B = BUNGY		
W = WHITE WATER PRACTICE	1 – 6 X 10 MIN	
RP = RACE PACE	1 – 6 X 10 MIN	UT
C = COURSE OR SIMILAR CONDITIONS		LSD
TREK/RUN		
E = EASY		
T = TECHNIQUE		
H = HILLS		
HH = REALLY BIG HILLS		
C = COURSE OR SIMILAR CONDITIONS		

GENERAL

FG = FULL GEAR
Do the workout with the weight of all your gear as this can have a big impact on how you operate and you comfort levels if you are unused to it. Also, use the gear you will use in the race (pack, clothing, socks, shoes) so everything is tested and proven and adjustments that need to be made have been carried out.
FS = FOOD SPECIFIC
Use the food that you will use in the event so as to get conditioned to it. Also, use these workouts to experiment with what works best for you and is easiest to use. (e.g. not too sticky, not too dry & crumbly)
N = NAVIGATION
Make sure that you are map reading and navigating during this workout. Ideally you want to do this in the type of conditions you expect for the event.
C = NAVIGATION TO CHECKPOINTS
As above but navigating to specific points on a map.
D = NIGHT WORKOUT
Do this workout at night to practice racing at night and to test all your lights and map reading.
SIM = SIMULATION
Simulations require a full dress rehearsal. This means that your whole team (in their roles), with the food you will use, wearing the gear you all will wear at apace half way between your usual training pace and race pace. Ideally this is performed in the environment and conditions you expect, with your support crew.
T = TEAM
Practice as a team
TP = TEMPO
Approx. max 8hr race race. 1 – 4 X 20 min

24-HOUR ADVENTURE RACE

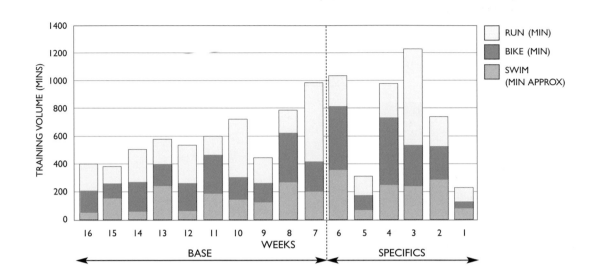

	16	15	14	13	12	11	10	9	8	7	6	5	4	3	2	1
WEEK	16	15	14	13	12	11	10	9	8	7	6	5	4	3	2	1
SUBPHASE	1+2	1+2	2	2	2	2+3	2+3	2+3	2+3	2+3	2+3	2+3	4+5	4+5	4+5	4+5
MESOCYCLE	Build	Recover	Build	Build	Recover	Build	Build	Recover	Build	Build	Build	Recover	Build	Build	Recover	Recover
TOTAL KAYAK	50	150	60	240	60	190	140	120	270	195	360	70	280	240	290	80
TIME BIKE	160	110	210	150	200	280	160	140	350	215	450	80	450	270	240	50
(MINS) TREK/RUN	190	130	240	190	280	130	420	190	170	570	220	160	240	720	210	100
MON KAYAK	20E+T	20E+T	30E+T	30E+T	30E	30E	40E	30E	50B	60B	70B	40E	80W	90W	60W	40E
MON BIKE																
MON RUN	30E+T	20E+T	30E+T	30E+T	30E+T	30H	30H	30E	40H	40H	60H	30E	60H	60H	60H	30E
TUES KAYAK																
TUES BIKE	40E+T	40E+T	50E+T	50H	40E	60H	60H	40E	60H	75H	90HH	40E	90RP	90RP	60RP	40E
TUES TREK																
WED KAYAK	30E	30E	30E	40E	30E	40E	40E	30E	40B	45B	50B	30E	60B	60B	50B	30E
WED BIKE																
WED TREK	40E	40E	50H	60H	40E	60H	70H	60E	80H	90H	100HH	90E	120HH	120HH	90H	60E
THURS KAYAK																
THURS BIKE	30E	30E	40H	40H	40E	40H	40H	40E	50HH	50HH	60HH	40E	60HH	60HH	60E	
THURS TREK	30H	30E	40H	40H	30E	40HH	40HH	40E	50RP	50RP	60RP	40E	60RP	60RP	60RP	
FRI KAYAK	ROPE DAY															10E
FRI BIKE	ROPE DAY															10E
FRI TREK	ROPE DAY															10E
SAT KAYAK		60E		90E		120E		60E	180E	FG/N	240E	SIM**	240E***	FG/FS	180E	RACE
SAT BIKE									60E	D			FG/FS	D/N		RACE
SAT TREK	90E		120E		180E		240H	60E	300HH				N	360HH		RACE
SUN KAYAK		40E		60E			60E	SIM*		90E		SIM**	D/N	90E		RACE
SUN BIKE	90E	40E	120E	60E	120E	180E	60E	N/FG	240E	90E	300HH	N/D/T	300H	120E	120E	RACE
SUN TREK		40E		60E			60E	D/T	FG/N	90E	FG/N	FS/FG	FG/FS	120E		RACE

NOTES :

Suggested Practice Events: 24hr Adventure Race Simulation in weeks 9 and 5

Rope Day: Practise all your rope work (e.g. abseiling) on this day.

Trekking: Asume for all trekking training that you use footwear, clothing and pack that will be used in the race.

KEY

	REPS	HR
BIKE		
E = EASY		LSD
T = TECHNIQUE		LSD
H = HILLS		
HH = REALLY BIG HILLS		
C = COURSE OR SIMILAR CONDITIONS		LSD
RP = RACE PACE	1 – 6 X 10 MIN	UT
KAYAK		
E = EASY		LSD
T = TECHNIQUE		LSD
B = BUNGY		
W = WHITE WATER PRACTICE	1 – 6 X 10 MIN	
RP = RACE PACE	1 – 6 X 10 MIN	UT
C = COURSE OR SIMILAR CONDITIONS		LSD
TREK/RUN		
E = EASY		LSD
T = TECHNIQUE		LSD
H = HILLS		
HH = REALLY BIG HILLS		
C = COURSE OR SIMILAR CONDITIONS		LSD
RP = RACE PACE	1 – 6 X 10 MIN	

GENERAL

FG = FULL GEAR
Do the workout with the weight of all your gear as this can have a big impact on how you operate and you comfort levels if you are unused to it. Also, use the gear you will use in the race (pack, clothing, socks, shoes) so everything is tested and proven and adjustments that need to be made have been carried out.
FS = FOOD SPECIFIC
Use the food that you will use in the event so as to get conditioned to it. Also, use these workouts to experiment with what works best for you and is easiest to use. (e.g. not too sticky, not too dry & crumbly)
N = NAVIGATION
Make sure that you are map reading and navigating during this workout. Ideally you want to do this in the type of conditions you expect for the event.
C = NAVIGATION TO CHECKPOINTS
As above but navigating to specific points on a map.
D = NIGHT WORKOUT
Do this workout at night to practice racing at night and to test all your lights and map reading.
SIM = SIMULATION
Simulations require a full dress rehearsal. This means that your whole team (in their roles), with the food you will use, wearing the gear you all will wear at apace half way between your usual training pace and race pace. Ideally this is performed in the environment and conditions you expect, with your support crew.
T = Team
Practise as a team

SWIMMING OPEN WATER RACE

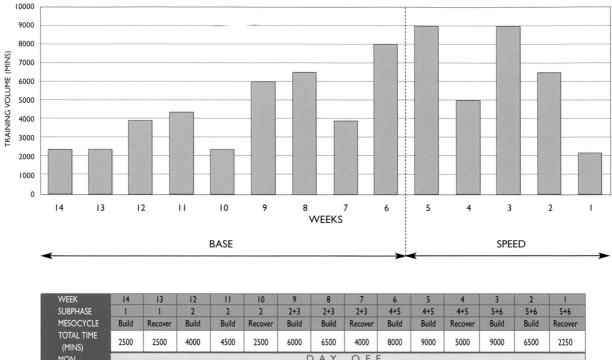

WEEK	14	13	12	11	10	9	8	7	6	5	4	3	2	1
SUBPHASE	1	1	2	2	2	2+3	2+3	2+3	4+5	4+5	4+5	5+6	5+6	5+6
MESOCYCLE	Build	Recover	Build	Build	Recover	Build	Build	Recover	Build	Build	Recover	Build	Build	Recover
TOTAL TIME (MINS)	2500	2500	4000	4500	2500	6000	6500	4000	8000	9000	5000	9000	6500	2250
MON	D A Y O F F													
TUES	500E+T	500E+T	1000PB	1000PB	500E	1000P	1000P	500E	1500RP	1500RP	1000E	1500RP	1500RP	1000E+C
WED	D A Y O F F													
THURS	500E+T	500E+T	1000E+T	1000PB	500E	1500PB	1500PB	1000E	2000PB	2000PB+P	1500E	2000PB+P	2000PB+P	1000E+C
FRI	D A Y O F F													
SAT	500E+T	500E+T	500A	500A	500E	1000UT	1000UT	500E	1000UT	1500UT	500E	1500A	1000UT	250E+C
SUN	1000E	1000E	1500E	2000E	1000E	2500E	3000E	2000E	3500E+C	4000E	2000E	4000UT+C	2000UT+C	EVENT

NOTES :

Suggested Practice Events: Open Water Race Simulation in weeks 8, 5 and 3
Pool Swimming: All training sessions marked in bold should be in the pool. All other sessions should be open water, if possible.

KEY		
	REPS	**HR**
SWIM		
E = EASY		LSD
T = TECHNIQUE		LSD
PB = PULL BUOY	1 – 5 X 200M	LSD
PD = PADDLES	1 – 8 X 50M	
RP = RACE PACE	1 – 6 X 1 MIN & 1 – 2 X 3 MIN	AT/UT
CO = CONTINUOUS		LSD
A = ACCELERATIONS	1 – 15 X 10-25M	UP TO AT
UT = UP TEMPO	1 – 6 X 33M	UT
C = COURSE OR SIMILAR CONDITIONS		LSD

ROWING AND KAYAKING TRAINING PROGRAMMES

16

Training notes

Land-based training

Starting with full on the water rowing training at the beginning of the season may not be effective in terms of the overall programme. Too much rowing will make you tire quickly early in the season and lose form. Therefore, the aim might be to start with a lot of land training and emphasise technique in 'on the water'.

Technique work is important in the early stages because it sets the technical rowing ability for the remainder of the season. Early season land training will have cardiovascular and muscular benefits without causing a deterioration in technique. The rowing training itself, which is technical in early season, will enhance rowing performance later on. This fits with the philosophy of doing base training first.

As you become fitter, more 'on the water' training occurs, with a gradual reduction in land-based training. Finally, towards the end of base training most, if not all, training is done 'on the water'. This gradual progression is ideal for both strength and technique.

Technique vs duration and intensity

In all sports with a technical component, the ability to perform the given task in a precise manner is crucial. Technique should not be sacrificed to tiredness, intensity or duration. It is commonly accepted that technique begins to deteriorate as you tire. Strategies to avoid this are:

1 Technique in target sport training followed by 'like-sport' training: Technique training should be followed by extra training in the 'like-sport' to boost muscular and cardiovascular fitness. Start with minimal target sport training, progressing as you become fitter and better able to maintain technique, to almost all target sport training.

   Always train in the target sport first, concentrating on technique while still 'fresh'. 'Like-sports' include rowing ergometer and rowing-specific gym exercises.
2 Split workouts: Training workouts are split up over a day, to minimise fatigue. The athlete splits training into shorter workouts in the morning and evening, with a recovery period in between.

Rowing in small boats at the beginning of the season

Using smaller boats at the beginning of the season (e.g. race in a coxless four but train in a pair) can be a very good way of improving technique – the smaller boats are a lot less forgiving on bad rowing technique. Later in the season, the key is to train the full crew in the type of boat (e.g. coxless four) in which they will race. At this point the coach can begin to mould the crew together to row as one unit.

Sport-specific training used for rowing

Type (intensity)	When initiated	Effect	Example
Power	Late speed phase	Faster, more powerful stroke	Starts, rest to recovery
Intensive sprints	Late speed phase	Improves starts and finishes	Extended start, 20–30 strokes
Extensive sprints	Speed phase	Improves extended starts and finishes	4–6 × 1–3 m rest to recovery
Submaximal btwn	Early speed phase	Improves max steady state race pace	4–6 × 6–8 m 4–1 min rest
Up-tempo pieces, btwn	Late base, early speed	Transition from base to speedwork	20–40 min rest to recovery
Long slow distance	Base/speed	Improves ability to do mileage, builds training tolerance and improves recovery rate	Continuous
Active	Base/speed	Assists recovery	Continuous

Proportions:
1 Base – 100% long slow distance and active recovery; some speedwork may be used.
2 Speed – approx. 85–90% long slow distance and active recovery; approx. 10–15% up-tempo and submaximal intensity.

RECREATIONAL 2000M ROWING RACE

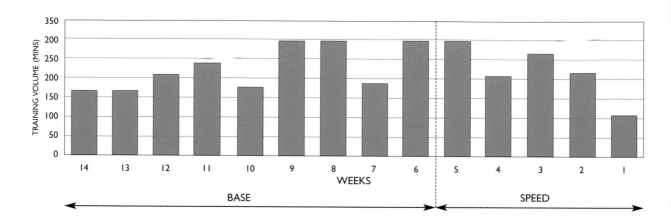

WEEK	14	13	12	11	10	9	8	7	6	5	4	3	2	1
SUBPHASE	1	1	2	2	2	2+3	2+3	2+3	4–6	4–6	4–6	6+7	6+7	6+7
MESOCYCLE	Build	Recover	Build	Build	Recover	Build	Build	Recover	Build	Build	Recover	Build	Build	Recover
TOTAL TIME (MINS)	170	170	210	240	180	300	300	190	300	300	210	270	220	110
MON					D A Y	O F F								
TUES	30E+T	30E+T	40SFP	40SFP	30E	40A	40A	30E	40RP	40RP	40E	30ST+A	40ST+A	30E
WED	30E+T	30E+T	40E+T	40E+T	40E+T	60B	60B	40E	50A	50A	30E	40RP	40RP	40A+C
THURS	40E+T	40E+T	50E+T	60SFP	40E	75SFP	75SFP	40E	60B	60B	40E	50B	40B	30ST+C
FRI					D A Y	O F F								
SAT	30E+T	30E+T	30B	40B	30E	50B	50B	40E	60ST	60ST	40E	60RP	40RP	10ST+C
SUN	40E+T	40E+T	50E+T	60E+T	40E+T	75SFP	75SFP	40E	90SFP	90SFP	60E	90SFP	60SFP	EVENT

NOTES :

Suggested Practice Events: Practice Regatta in weeks 8, 7, 4 and 2

KEY			
		REPS	HR
ROWING			
E = EASY			LSD
T = TECHNIQUE			LSD
SFP = SLOW FULL PRESSURE		1 – 6 X 10 MIN	LSD
B = BUNGY		1 – 4 X 10 MIN	
ST = STARTS		1 – 6	
RP = RACE PACE		1 – 6 X 1 MIN & 1 – 2 X 3 MIN	AT/HI
A = ACCELERATIONS		1 – 10 X 30S	UP TO AT
C = COURSE OR SIMILAR CONDITIONS			LSD

RECREATIONAL KAYAK RACE

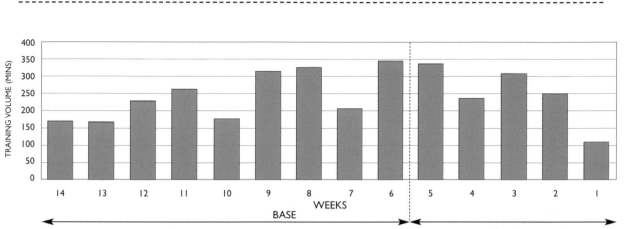

WEEK	14	13	12	11	10	9	8	7	6	5	4	3	2	1
SUBPHASE	1	1	2	2	2	2+3	2+3	2+3	4-6	4-6	4-6	6+7	6+7	6+7
MESOCYCLE	Build	Recover	Build	Build	Recover	Build	Build	Recover	Build	Build	Recover	Build	Build	Recover
TOTAL TIME (MINS)	170	170	230	265	180	320	330	210	350	340	240	310	250	110
MON	D A Y O F F													
TUES	30E+T	30E+T	40SFP	40SFP	30E	40A	40A	30E	40RP	40RP	40E	30ST+A	40ST+A	30E
WED	30E+T	30E+T	40E+T	40E+T	40E+T	60B	60B	40E	50A	50A	30E	40RP	40RP	40A+C
THURS	40E+T	40E+T	60E+T	75SFP	40E	90SFP	90SFP	40E	80B	70B	40E	60B	40B	30ST+C
FRI	D A Y O F F													
SAT	30E+T	30E+T	30B	40B	30E	50B	50B	40E	60ST	60ST	40E	60RP	40RP	10ST+C
SUN	40E+T	40E+T	60E+T	70E+T	40E+T	80SFP	100SFP	60E	120SFP	120SFP	90E	120SFP	90SFP	EVENT

NOTES :

Suggested Practice Events: Kayak Race Simulation in weeks 7, 4 and 2

KEY		
	REPS	**HR**
KAYAKING		
E = EASY		LSD
T = TECHNIQUE		LSD
SFP = SLOW FULL PRESSURE	1 – 6 X 10 MIN	LSD
B = BUNGY	1 – 4 X 10 MIN	
ST = STARTS	1 – 6	
RP = RACE PACE	1 – 6 X 1 MIN &	AT/UT
	1 – 2 X 3 MIN	
A = ACCELERATIONS	1 – 10 X 30S	UP TO AT
C = COURSE OR SIMILAR CONDITIONS		LSD

ROAD CYCLING TRAINING PROGRAMMES

17

Training notes for road cycling

Spinning, cadence and gear selection in base training

Many cyclists tend to start their build-up by pushing big gears at a slow cadence, for example 65–80 rpm. This can cause stress on the knees and injuries may occur. It is more beneficial to start in a very easy gear, such as 42 ´ 18, and maintain a high rpm. 85–95 rpm is an optimal time trial cadence for triathletes; 90–110 is good for cyclists and mountain bikers. These cadences will help prevent injury, and improve fitness, pedalling fluidity and technique. Bigger gears will be used later in the season when the body can tolerate the load.

Spinning is very important for a number of reasons. It allows you to sprint quickly if another cyclist tries to jump. In a big gear at low rpm it is harder to respond quickly. At high rpm, however, the response can be much quicker and the acceleration needed to match the jump can be achieved rapidly. Spinning in a smaller gear means you can change to a bigger gear as you build up speed following the jump.

Spinning is also good for conserving strength. Pushing big gears is much harder work than pushing the equivalent loads at higher rpms. If you push too high a gear, you may find that towards the end of the race you have tired legs. As a result you may fall behind on a hill or lose the sprint despite being fit enough to stay with the bunch right up to the final 200–300 metres.

Possible gearing in pre-season

Base 1 (6 weeks)
2 weeks: 42 ´ 18+ (only). This limits leg fatigue, helps prevent injury, increases fitness and improves pedalling technique.
2 weeks: 42 ´ 16+ (only).
2 weeks: Open gears but still use planned cadence: 85–95 rpm for triathletes and 90–110 rpm for cyclists.

Base 2 and Speed
Open gears, maintain optimal cadence in all rides. *Note:* In Base 2 and speed phases, limit easy rides to smaller gears to aid recovery; all easy rides 42 ´ 16+ only.

Cycle tours vs single-day cycle races

The major training emphasis for tours is mileage. If you are going to be racing 500 km in four days, or 900 km in a week, you need to be able to do this in training. Peak-mileage weeks for tours are very different to those for single-day races. For tours, the peak mileages are much higher and they are maintained approximately up until the last four weeks before the race. (Some cyclists use another tour as a warm-up.) For single-day racing, peak mileages are smaller and occur further away from race day (four to eight weeks) as more speedwork is required between base and peak. Too many single-day cyclists maintain mileage too close to the race. This leaves them slow (not enough speedwork) and fatigued.

Approximate timing of peak mileage

Long tours (more than a week): two to four weeks before peak race; short tours (less than a week): three to four weeks before peak race; 160 km race: four to six weeks before peak race; 40–80 km: six to eight weeks before peak race.

All off road rides are measured by time as it is difficult to determine distance off road.

Sport-specific training used for road cycling

Type (intensity)	When initiated	Effect	Example
Power	Late speed phase	Improves jump accels	4–6 × 10–15 sec rest to recovery
Intensive sprints	Late speed phase	Improves full sprint phase	6–10 × 30 sec–1 min rest to recovery or short rest < 1 min
Extensive sprints	Speed phase	Improves long sprint bridging gaps	4–6 × 1–3 min rest to recovery or 1–2 min btwn
Submaximal	Speed phase	Improves max steady state pace in TTs peloton and breaks	4–6 × 6–8 min 4–1 min rest btwn or 20–30 min TT
Up-tempo	Late base, early speed	Transition from base to speedwork	1–2 × 5–10 km rest 5 km btwn
Long slow distance	Base/speed	Improves ability to do mileage, builds training tolerance and improves recovery rate	Continuous
Active recovery	Base/speed	Assists recovery	Continuous

Proportions:
1 Base – 100% long slow distance and active recovery; some speedwork may be used.
2 Speed – approx. 85–90% long slow distance and active recovery; approx. 10–15% submaximal intensity and higher intensities.

RECREATIONAL 40KM ROAD RACE

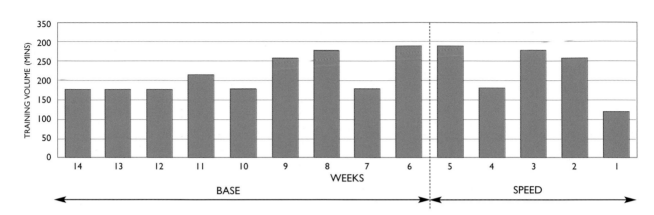

WEEK	14	13	12	11	10	9	8	7	6	5	4	3	2	1
SUBPHASE	1	1	2	2	2	2/3	2/3	2/3	4–6	4–6	4–6	7–9	7–9	7–9
MESOCYCLE	Build	Recover	Build	Build	Recover	Build	Build	Recover	Build	Build	Recover	Build	Build	Recover
TOTAL TIME (MINS)	180	180	180	215	180	255	280	180	290	290	180	280	255	120
MON	D A Y O F F													
TUES	40H	40E	40H	40H+Hbg	40E	60H+Hbg	60Fbg	40E	60S	60S	40E	60SP+A	60SP+A	40SP+A
WED	D A Y O F F													
THURS	40E	40E	40E	60H	40E	60H	70H+Hbg	40E	80H+Hbg	80H+Hbg	40E	70H+Hbg	60H+Hbg	40E+C
FRI	D A Y O F F													
SAT	40E+T	40E+T	40E+T	40E+T	40E	60A	60A	40E	60A	60A	40E	60S	60S	40E+C
SUN	60E	60E	60E	75H	60E	75H	90H	60E+C	90Fbg+C	90Fbg	60E+C	90Fbg+C	75E+C	EVENT

NOTES :

Suggested Practice Events: 40km Cycle Road Race in weeks 8, 5 and 3

Bunch Riding: Try to incorporate lots of bunch riding into your training

KEY		
	REPS	**HR**
BIKE		
E = EASY		LSD
T = TECHNIQUE		LSD
H = HILLS		
HBG = HILLS BIG GEAR	1 – 3 X 500M	
FBG = FLAT BIG GEAR	1 – 4 X 10 MIN	
RP = RACE PACE	1 – 2 X 5 MIN	AT
A = ACCELERATIONS	1 – 10 X 30S	UP TO AT
SP = SPRINT	1 – 4 X 200M	
C = COURSE OR SIMILAR CONDITIONS		LSD

RECREATIONAL 100KM ROAD RACE

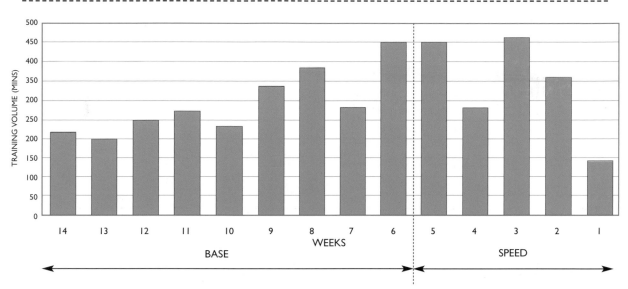

WEEK	14	13	12	11	10	9	8	7	6	5	4	3	2	1
SUBPHASE	1	1	2	2	2	2+3	2+3	2+3	4–6	4–6	4–6	7–9	7–9	7–9
MESOCYCLE	Build	Recover	Build	Build	Recover	Build	Build	Recover	Build	Build	Recover	Build	Build	Recover
TOTAL TIME (MINS)	220	200	250	270	230	335	385	280	450	450	280	460	355	140
MON	D A Y O F F													
TUES	40H	40E	60H	60H+Hbg	40E	75H+Hbg	75Fbg	60E	90RP	90RP	60E	90SP+A	75SP+A	60SP+A
WED	D A Y O F F													
THURS	60E	60E	70E	80H	60E	80H	100H+Hbg	90E	120H+Hbg	120H+Hbg	60E	120H+Hbg	100H+Hbg	40E+C
FRI	D A Y O F F													
SAT	40E+T	40E+T	40E+T	40E+T	40E	60A	60A	40E	60A	60A	40E	60RP	60RP	40E+C
SUN	80E	60E	80E	100H	90E	120H	150H	90E+C	180Fbg+C	180Fbg	120E+C	180Fbg+C	120E+C	EVENT

NOTES :

Suggested Practice Events: 100km Cycle Road Race in weeks 8, 5 and 3

Club Racing: Weekly club racing is recommended but use the suggested practice events as an opportunity to race more seriously

Speedwork: If club racing, remove speedwork. If you do wish to do speedwork, make sure that you use the correct intensities. Speedwork at the wrong intensity will not be beneficial for your training.

KEY			
		REPS	HR
BIKE			
E = EASY			LSD
T = TECHNIQUE			LSD
H = HILLS			
HBG = HILLS BIG GEAR		1 – 3 X 500M	
FBG = FLAT BIG GEAR		1 – 4 X 10 MIN	
RP = RACE PACE		1 – 2 X 5 MIN	AT/UT
A = ACCELERATIONS		1 – 10 X 30S	UP TO AT
SP = SPRINT		1 – 4 X 200M	
C = COURSE OR SIMILAR CONDITIONS			LSD

ADVANCED 100KM ROAD RACE

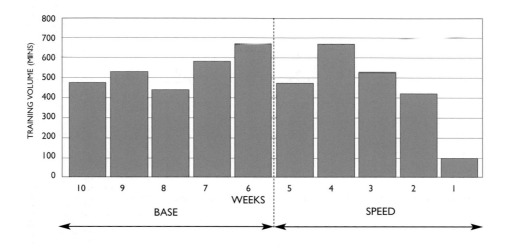

NOTES :

Suggested Practice Events: Bunch race on Thursday of every week

For more information, please refer to the Detailed Training Programme Keys
on pp. 214–222

WEEK	10	9	8	7	6	5	4	3	2	1	REPS	HEART RATE
SUBPHASE	2	2	2	3+4	3+4	3+4	5+6	5+6	7–9	7–9		
MESOCYCLE	BUILD	BUILD	RECOVER	BUILD	BUILD	RECOVER	BUILD	RECOVER	BUILD	RECOVER		
TOTAL	480	540	450	590	680	480	680	540	420	100		
MON	60	60	60	60	60	60	60	60	60	30	REPS	HEART RATE
OSPD							1 SPT	2 SPT	2 SPT	1 SPT	REPS X 200M	N/A
P/S	1 PWR	2 PWR	1 PWR	3 PWR	2 PWR	1 PWR	1 PWR	1 PWR	1 PWR	1 PWR	REPS X 200M	N/A
DRILLS											DO DRILLS	N/A
ACC/CR	2	3	2	3	4	2	5	2	4	1	REPS X 30SECS	UP TO AT
FUT											REPS X 10MINS	UT
FBG											REPS X 20MINS	LSD
LC/TC											REPS X 10MINS	N/A
H/Hs											ALL	N/A
TERR	RH	RH	F	RH	RH	F	F	F	F	RH	N/A	
TUES	60	60	60	80	80	60	80	60	60	20		
OSPD	HILL CLMB	HILL CLMB	HILL CLMB	HILL CLMB	HILL CLMB	HILL CLMB	HILL CLMB	HILL CLMB	HILL CLMB		REPS X 200M	N/A
P/S											REPS X 200M	N/A
DRILLS											DO DRILLS	N/A
ACC/CR	1 CR	1 CR	1 CR	1 CR	2 CR	1 CR	2 CR	3 CR	3 CR	2	REPS X 30SECS	UP TO AT
FUT										1	REPS X 10MINS	UT
FBG											REPS X 20MINS	LSD
LC/TC	2 LC	3 LC	1 LC	3 LC	4LC	1 LC	2 TC	1LC	2 TC		REPS X 10MINS	N/A
H/Hs											ALL	N/A
TERR	H	H	RH	H	H	RH	H	RH	H	F	N/A	
WED	60	60	60	60	60	60	60	60	60	30		
OSPD										1	REPS X 200M	N/A
P/S										1 PWR	REPS X 200M	N/A
DRILLS	DRILLS	DRILLS	DRILLS	DRILLS	DRILLS	DRILLS	DRILLS	DRILLS	DRILLS		DO DRILLS	N/A
ACC/CR										2	REPS X 30SECS	UP TO AT
FUT							2	2	2	1	REPS X 10MINS	UT
FBG	2		1	2	3	1	1	1	1		REPS X 20MINS	LSD
LC/TC											REPS X 10MINS	N/A
H/Hs											ALL	N/A
TERR	RH	RH	F	RH	RH	F	RH	F	RH	F	N/A	
THURS	60	60	60	60	60	60	60	60	60			
OSPD	BUNCH	BUNCH	BUNCH	BUNCH	BUNCH	BUNCH	BUNCH	BUNCH	BUNCH		REPS X 200M	N/A
P/S	(SIT IN)	(SIT IN)	(SIT IN)	(SIT IN)	(SIT IN)	(STIR)	(RACE)	(STIR)	(RACE)		REPS X 200M	N/A
DRILLS											DO DRILLS	N/A
ACC/CR	START	START		START	START						REPS X 30SECS	UP TO AT
FUT	FRESH	FRESH	FRESH	TOP 1/3	TOP 1/3	TOP 1/3	CONTEST	TOP 1/3	CONTEST		REPS X 10MINS	UT
FBG											REPS X 20MINS	LSD
LC/TC	W/UP	W/UP	W/UP	W/UP	W/UP	W/UP	W/UP	W/UP	W/UP		REPS X 10MINS	N/A
H/Hs	TECH	TECH	TECH	TECH	TECH	TECH	TECH	TECH	TECH		ALL	N/A
TERR												
FRI										20		
OSPD										1	REPS X 200M	N/A
P/S										1 PWR	REPS X 200M	N/A
DRILLS											DO DRILLS	N/A
ACC/CR										2	REPS X 30SECS	UP TO AT
FUT										1	REPS X 10MINS	UT
FBG											REPS X 20MINS	LSD
LC/TC											REPS X 10MINS	N/A
H/Hs											ALL	N/A
TERR												
SAT	120	150	90	150	180	120	180	120	60	100KM		
OSPD			COURSE		1 SPT		COURSE		2 SPT		REPS X 200M	N/A
P/S	2 PWR				3 PWR				4 PWR		REPS X 200M	N/A
DRILLS	BUNCH				BUNCH				BUNCH		DO DRILLS	N/A
ACC/CR		RACING		RACING		RACING		RACING			REPS X 30SECS	UP TO AT
FUT		DRILLS		DRILLS		DRILLS		DRILLS			REPS X 10MINS	UT
FBG	2				4				2		REPS X 20MINS	LSD
LC/TC											REPS X 10MINS	N/A
H/Hs											ALL	N/A
TERR												
SUN	120	150	120	180	240	120	240	180	120			
OSPD											REPS X 200M	N/A
P/S											REPS X 200M	N/A
DRILLS	BUNCH	BUNCH	BUNCH	BUNCH	BUNCH	BUNCH	BUNCH	BUNCH	BUNCH		DO DRILLS	N/A
ACC/CR	4	6	3	9	12	4	16	6	4		REPS X 30SECS	UP TO AT
FUT											REPS X 10MINS	UT
FBG			2		3		2				REPS X 20MINS	LSD
LC/TC	1 LC	2 LC		3 LC	6 LC		2 LC		2 LC		REPS X 10MINS	N/A
H/Hs											ALL	N/A
TERR	H	H	RH	H	H	RH	RH	RH	RH		N/A	

RECREATIONAL 160KM ROAD RACE

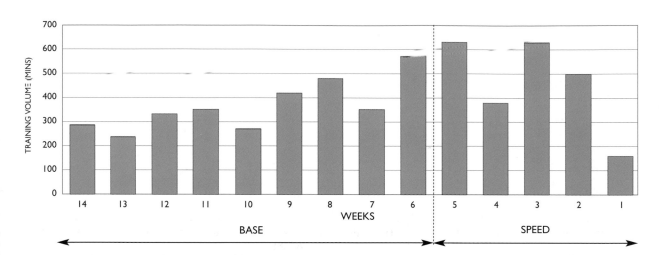

WEEK	14	13	12	11	10	9	8	7	6	5	4	3	2	1
SUBPHASE	1	1	2	2	2	2+3	2+3	2+3	4–6	4–6	4–6	7–9	7–9	7–9
MESOCYCLE	Build	Recover	Build	Build	Recover	Build	Build	Recover	Build	Build	Recover	Build	Build	Recover
TOTAL TIME (MINS)	290	240	330	350	270	420	480	350	570	630	380	630	490	160
MON	DAY OFF													
TUES	40H	40E	60H	60H+Hbg	40E	60H+Hbg	60Fbg	40E	60S	60S	40E	60SP+A	60SP+A	60SP+A
WED	60E	40E	60E	60E	40E	70E	80E	60E	90E	90E	60E	90FUT	90FUT	D/O
THURS	60E	60E	70E	80H	60E	80H	100H+Hbg	90E	120H+Hbg	120H+Hbg	60E	120H+Hbg	100H+Hbg	40E+C
FRI	DAY OFF													
SAT	40E+T	40E+T	40E+T	40E+T	40E	60A	60A	40E	60A	60A	40E	60S	60S	40E+C
SUN	90E	60E	100E	120H	90E	150H	180H	120E+C	240Fbg+C	300Fbg	180E+C	300Fbg+C	180E+C	EVENT

NOTES :

Suggested Practice Events: 160km Bike Race Simulation in weeks 7, 4 and 3

Bunch Riding: Try to do lots of bunch riding

KEY		
	REPS	**HR**
BIKE		
E = EASY		LSD
T = TECHNIQUE		LSD
H = HILLS		
HBG = HILLS BIG GEAR	1 – 3 X 500M	
FBG = FLAT BIG GEAR	1 – 4 X 10 MIN	
FUT = FLAT BIG GEAR UP TEMPO	1 – 4 X 10 MIN	UT
S = SPEED	1 – 2 X 5 MIN	AT
RP = RACE PACE	1 – 2 X 5 MIN	UT
A = ACCELERATIONS	1 – 10 X 30S	UP TO AT
SP = SPRINT	1 – 4 X 200M	
C = COURSE OR SIMILAR CONDITIONS		LSD

RECREATIONAL 160KM DOUBLE BUILD UP

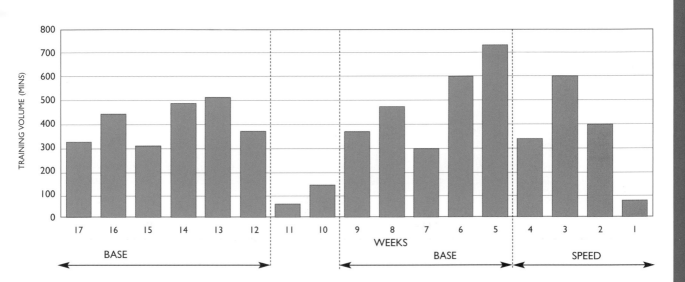

WEEK	17	16	15	14	13	12	11	10	9	8	7	6	5	4	3	2	1
SUBPHASE	2+3	2+3	2+3	2–4	2–4	2–4			2–4	2–4	2–4	5+6	5+6	5+6	7–9	7–9	7–9
MESOCYCLE	Build	Build	Recover	Build	Build	Recover	Recover	Recover	Build	Build	Build	Recover	Build	Recover	Build	Build	Recover
EFFORT	DILIGENT				FOCUS		REST		RELAX			DILIGENT			FOCUS		
TOTAL TIME (MINS)	330	450	310	500	520	380	60	140	370	480	300	600	750	340	600	400	70
MON	DAY OFF																
TUES	40H/Hs	60H/LC	40RH	60H/LC	60H/LC	40RH			40H	60H/LC	40RH	60RH/A	90RH/A	40RP/P	60RP/P	60RP/P	30
WED	30FBG	40FBG		40FBG/A	40FBG/A		20E	20E	40FBG	60FBG		80FBG	60FBG/A		40FUT	40FUT	20E
THURS	60H/Hs	80H/Hs	90RH	100H/Hs	120H/Hs	20RH			60H/LC	80H/LC	60E	100H/LC	120H/TC	60RH	80H/TC	60RH	
FRI																	20E
SAT	80FUT	120H/LC	60RH	120H/LC	60R	20E			80FBG	100FBG/A	80E	120R	180R	60RH	120R	180R	160KM
SUN	120H/Hs	150H/Hs	120B/RH	180B/RH	240B/RH	300H	40E	120E	150B/RH	180B/RH	120RH	240B/RH	300RH	180RH/LC	300RH	60RH	

NOTES :

Suggested Practice Events: Races in weeks 7, 4 and 3

Bunch Riding: Try to incorporate lots of bunch riding into your training

KEY		
	REPS	**HR**
BIKE		
E = EASY		
T = TECHNIQUE		
H = HILLS		
HS = HILLS SPIN		
FBG = FLAT BIG GEAR	1 – 3 X 20 MIN	
R = CLUB RACE		
A = ACCELERATIONS		
SP = SPRINT	1 – 4 X 200M	
P = POWER	1 – 2 X 200M	
LC = LONG CLIMBS	1 – 3 X 10 MIN	
TC = TEMPO CLIMBS	1 – 3 X 10 MIN	
B = BUNCH RIDE		
C = COURSE OR SIMILAR CONDITIONS		
RP = RACE PACE	1 – 2 X 5MIN	AT

ADVANCED 160KM ROAD RACE

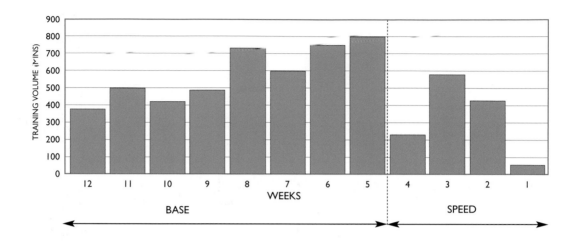

NOTES :

Rest Weeks : You should have one complete rest week before starting this programme

For more information, please refer to the Detailed Training Programme Keys on pp. 214–222

	12	11	10	9	8	7	6	5	4	3	2	1	REPS	HEART RATE
WEEK	12	11	10	9	8	7	6	5	4	3	2	1		
SUBPHASE	2+3	2+3	2+3	2-4	2-4	2-4	5+6	5+6	7-9	7-9	7-9	7-9		
MESOCYCLE	BUILD	BUILD	RECOVER	BUILD	BUILD	RECOVER	BUILD	BUILD	RECOVER	BUILD	BUILD	RECOVER		
TOTAL	390	510	430	500	740	600	760	800	240	590	440	60		
EFFORT		RELAX					DILIGENT			FOCUS				
MON														
O/S & CR													REPS X 200M	N/A
PWR & SPT													REPS X 200M	N/A
UT													REPS X 10MINS	UT
ACC													REPS X 30SECS	UP TO AT
FUT													REPS X 10MINS	UT
FBG													REPS X 20MINS	LSD
LC/TC													REPS X 10MINS	N/A
H/Hs													ALL	N/A
TERR													N/A	
TUES	40	60	40	60	80	40	80	80	40	60	60	40		
O/S & CR		2 CR	1 SPT	3 CR	4 CR			1 SPT	2 PWR	1 PWR			REPS X 200M	N/A
PWR & SPT		1 PWR	1 PWR	1 PWR	1 PWR	2 PWR	3 PWR	4 PWR	2 SPT	3 SPT	4 SPT	1 SPT	REPS X 200M	N/A
UT													REPS X 10MINS	UT
ACC	2	4	2	4	6	2	6	8	2	8	8	2	REPS X 30SECS	UP TO AT
FUT													REPS X 10MINS	UT
FBG													REPS X 20MINS	LSD
LC/TC		2 LC		3 LC	3 LC								REPS X 10MINS	N/A
H/Hs		Hs		Hs	Hs								ALL	N/A
TERR	H	HH	RH	HH	HH	RH	RH	RH	F	F	F	F	N/A	
WED	60	80	40	80	90	40	80	90	60	60	60			
O/S & CR									RACE	RACE	RACE		REPS X 200M	N/A
PWR & SPT									AGITATE	SIT IN	AGITATE		REPS X 200M	N/A
UT													REPS X 10MINS	UT
ACC	4	6	6	6	8	4	6	6					REPS X 30SECS	UP TO AT
FUT				1	2		3	4					REPS X 10MINS	UT
FBG	2	4		1	1	2	1						REPS X 20MINS	LSD
LC/TC													REPS X 10MINS	N/A
H/Hs													ALL	N/A
TERR	RH	RH			RH	F	RH		F	F	F		N/A	
THURS	80	100	80	120	150	120	120	150	120	90	80			
O/S & CR		1 CR		2 CR	2 CR		2 CR	2 CR		2 CR	2 CR		REPS X 200M	N/A
PWR & SPT													REPS X 200M	N/A
UT													REPS X 10MINS	UT
ACC													REPS X 30SECS	UP TO AT
FUT													REPS X 10MINS	UT
FBG										2 LC	1 LC		REPS X 20MINS	LSD
LC/TC		1 LC		2 LC	3 LC	1 LC	3 LC	4 LC	1 LC	1 TC	1 TC		REPS X 10MINS	N/A
H/Hs	Hs	Hs		Hs	Hs		Hs	Hs					ALL	N/A
TERR	H	HH	H	HH	HH	RH	H	HH	RH	H	H		N/A	
FRI											20			
O/S & CR											1 O/S		REPS X 200M	N/A
PWR & SPT											1 SPT		REPS X 200M	N/A
UT													REPS X 10MINS	UT
ACC											2		REPS X 30SECS	UP TO AT
FUT											1		REPS X 10MINS	UT
FBG													REPS X 20MINS	LSD
LC/TC													REPS X 10MINS	N/A
H/Hs													ALL	N/A
TERR											F		N/A	
SAT	90	120	150	60	180	40	180	120	20	80	60			
O/S & CR							RACE	RACE	1 O/S	RACE	RACE		REPS X 200M	N/A
PWR & SPT		1 PWR	1 SPT	2 PWR	2 PWR	1 SPT	SIT IN	AGITATE	1 SPT	AGITATE	SIT IN		REPS X 200M	N/A
UT													REPS X 10MINS	UT
ACC	4	6	1	8	10	2			2				REPS X 30SECS	UP TO AT
FUT	1	2		3	4	1			1				REPS X 10MINS	UT
FBG													REPS X 20MINS	LSD
LC/TC													REPS X 10MINS	N/A
H/Hs													ALL	N/A
TERR	H	H	F		F	F	RH	RH	F	F	F		N/A	
SUN	120	150	120	180	240	360	300	360	RACE	300	180			
O/S & CR	1 CR	2 CR	3 CR	1 CR	BUNCH	COURSE	2 CR	BUNCH	OR	BUNCH	BUNCH		REPS X 200M	N/A
PWR & SPT					SIT IN	CHECK		SIT IN	120KM	SIT IN	TEMPO		REPS X 200M	N/A
UT									TEMPO				REPS X 10MINS	UT
ACC									BUNCH				REPS X 30SECS	UP TO AT
FUT									RIDE				REPS X 10MINS	UT
FBG													REPS X 20MINS	LSD
LC/TC	2 LC	3 LC	2 LC	4 LC			4 LC						REPS X 10MINS	N/A
H/Hs		Hs	Hs	Hs			Hs						ALL	N/A
TERR	H	HH	HH	HH	RH		H	RH	RH	RH	RH		N/A	

273

2–3 DAY CYCLE TOUR

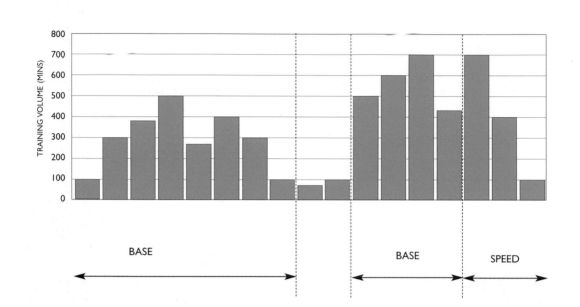

NOTES :

Suggested Practice Events: 100–160km Road Race in week 10
Training races on Saturday of weeks 14, 13, 11, 6, 4, 3 and 2

Rest Weeks: You should have 4 weeks of complete rest before starting this training programme

Key Weeks: Weeks 14, 12, 5, and 3 are shaded to emphasise that these are your key training weeks

Key Workouts: Key workouts are represented by dark shading

WEEK	16	15	14	13	12	11	10	9	8	7	6	5	4	3	2	1	REPS	HEART RATE
MESOCYCLE	H	H	H	E	H	H	E	E	E	H	H	H	E	H	H	E		
TOTAL	300	400	510	280	410	300	80	70	100	510	620	720	440	720	410	120		
MON																	REPS	HEART RATE
O/S & CR																	REPS X 200M	N/A
PW & SPT																	REPS X 200M	N/A
UT																	REPS X 10MINS	UT
ACC																	REPS X 30SECS	UP TO AT
FUT																	REPS X 10MINS	UT
FBG																	REPS X 20MINS	LSD
LC/TC																	REPS X 10MINS	N/A
H/Hs																	ALL	N/A
TERR																		N/A
TUES	60	60	60	40	60	60	40			120	120	120	60	120	90	60		
O/S & CR		BGTT	BGTT	1 SPT	BGTT	BGTT	1 SPT			1 SPT	BGTT	BGTT	1 SPT	BGTT	3 SPT	2 SPT	REPS X 200M	N/A
PW & SPT		70RPM	70RPM	2 PWR	75RPM	80RPM	2 PWR			2 PWR	70RPM	75RPM	4 PWR	80RPM	2 PWR	2 PWR	REPS X 200M	N/A
UT		10KM	10KM		10KM	10KM					10KM	10KM		10KM			REPS X 10MINS	N/A
ACC				3 ACC			3 ACC			3 ACC			2 ACC		4 ACC	2 ACC	REPS X 30SECS	UP TO AT
FUT																	REPS X 10MINS	UT
FBG	2																REPS X 20MINS	LSD
LC/TC																	REPS X 10MINS	N/A
H/Hs																	ALL	N/A
TERR																		N/A
	20E	20E	20E	20E	20E	20E	20E			10E	10E	10E	30E	10E	20E			
WED							20	30	40	60	80	60	60	60	60	40		
O/S & CR							1 PWR			1 CR	2 CR		2 CR	3 CR		1 PWR	REPS X 200M	N/A
PW & SPT							1 SPT									1 SPT	REPS X 200M	N/A
UT																	REPS X 10MINS	N/A
ACC							1									1	REPS X 30SECS	UP TO AT
FUT							1									1	REPS X 10MINS	UT
FBG																	REPS X 20MINS	LSD
LC/TC										2 LC	4 LC	3 LC					REPS X 10MINS	N/A
H/Hs																	ALL	N/A
TERR										H	H	H		RH	RH			N/A
	20H	20H/He	30H/He	20A	30RH/A	30RH/A				20H/He	30H/He	30H/He	20A	20H/He	20A	20A		
THURS	80	100	120	60	80	60				120	120				60			
O/S & CR	W/UP 20	W/UP 20	W/UP 20	W/UP 20	W/UP 20	W/UP 20							W/UP 20		W/UP 20		REPS X 200M	N/A
PW & SPT	FBG30	FBG40	FBG50	FBG30	FBG30	FBG30							FBG30		FBG30		REPS X 200M	N/A
UT	TT3KM	TT3KM	TT4KM	TT3KM	TT4KM	TT5KM							TT4KM		TT4KM		REPS X 10MINS	N/A
ACC	W/DOWN	W/DOWN	W/DOWN	W/DOWN	W/DOWN	W/DOWN							W/DOWN		W/DOWN		REPS X 30SECS	UP TO AT
FUT																	REPS X 10MINS	UT
FBG																	REPS X 20MINS	LSD
LC/TC										2 LC	3 LC						REPS X 10MINS	N/A
H/Hs											Hs	Hs					ALL	N/A
TERR											H	H						N/A
	10E	20E	10E	20E	20E	10E				10E	10E		10E		10E			
FRI							20					120		120		20		
O/S & CR							1 PWR					2 CR				1 PWR	REPS X 200M	N/A
PW & SPT				1 SPT										1 SPT			REPS X 200M	N/A
UT																	REPS X 10MINS	N/A
ACC							1									1	REPS X 30SECS	UP TO AT
FUT							1									1	REPS X 10MINS	UT
FBG																	REPS X 20MINS	LSD
LC/TC												4 LC		2 LC			REPS X 10MINS	N/A
H/Hs												Hs		Hs			ALL	N/A
TERR												H		RH				N/A
SAT	40	60	90	60	90	60	RACE			90	120	180	80	180	80	TOUR		
O/S & CR	FBG	FBG	RACE	RACE	FBG	RACE					RACE		RACE	RACE	RACE		REPS X 200M	N/A
PW & SPT	ALL	ALL	SIT IN	RACE	ALL	SIT IN					SIT IN		SIT IN	RACE	SIT IN		REPS X 200M	N/A
UT	RIDE	RIDE			RIDE												REPS X 10MINS	N/A
ACC																	REPS X 30SECS	UP TO AT
FUT																	REPS X 10MINS	UT
FBG																	REPS X 20MINS	LSD
LC/TC												2 LC					REPS X 10MINS	N/A
H/Hs												Hs					ALL	N/A
TERR												H						N/A
	20E	30RH	30RH	20E	30RH	20E		20E	20E	30E	30E	40E	20E	30E	30E			
SUN	120	180	240	120	180	120	40	60		120	180	240	180	240	120	TOUR		
O/S & CR		1 CR		2 CR		2 CR				1 CR	2 CR		2 CR		1 CR		REPS X 200M	N/A
PW & SPT	BUNCH			BUNCH		BUNCH				BUNCH	BUNCH		BUNCH		BUNCH		REPS X 200M	N/A
UT																	REPS X 10MINS	N/A
ACC																	REPS X 30SECS	UP TO AT
FUT																	REPS X 10MINS	UT
FBG																	REPS X 20MINS	LSD
LC/TC	2 LC	3 LC	4 LC	1 TC	2 TC	1 TC				2 LC	3 LC	2 TC	4 LC	1 TC			REPS X 10MINS	N/A
H/Hs		Hs	Hs		Hs						Hs		Hs				ALL	N/A
TERR	RH	H	H	RH	H	RH				RH	RH	H	RH	H	RH			N/A

MOUNTAIN BIKING TRAINING PROGRAMMES

18

Mountain biking is cycling using bikes specially designed for off-road conditions. This usually means wider profile tyres, a stronger, more compact frame, more gears and shocks. Mountain biking has opened up training and competing in the outdoors and the mountain bike has become the bike of choice for most cycle buyers. Races are often short (1–3 hours) and involve technical trail riding – cross-country mountain biking. More demanding races are multi-day stage races – held in locations such as the European Alps, the Rockies and even in the desert. There are other forms of mountain biking, such as downhill racing which depends on the rider being very brave and technically skilled.

The key things to remember are:

1. The start. You will need to be prepared for a fast start. Competitive riders will try to get to the narrower parts of the course ahead of others. If you get stuck behind at this point there will be too much traffic to let you go fast.

2. Improve your single track and downhill skills. Find a single track or downhill stretch and try doing repeated intervals. This will allow you to hone your ability and speed in a measurable way. Repeat this till you feel you have mastered the section and then move on to another more technical stretch of track.

3. Practice running, mounting, dismounting and carrying your bike for obstacles.

4. Ride 'off road' about 3 times a week and ride on the road the rest of the time. Too much 'off road' will cause fatigue over a few months.

5. Mountain biking follows a 'surge and roll' pattern. Mountain biking is really a series of surges followed by rolling where you negotiate a technical aspect of the terrain. Most mountain bikers focus too much on continuous effort and cadence riding and are not prepared for the racing.

6. Downhill sections are not for resting – keep working!

7. Hills, hills, hills. There is a reason why it's called mountain biking!

Sport-specific training used in mountain biking

Type (intensity)	When initiated	Effect	Example
Power	–	–	–
Intensive sprints	–	–	–
Extensive sprints	Speed phase	Improves short hill climbs and starts	4–6 x 1–3 min rest to recovery or 1–2 min btwn
Submaximal	Speed phase	Improves max steady state pace for racing	4–6 x 6–8 min 4–1 min rest btwn or 20–30 min TT
Up-tempo	Late base, early speed	Transition from base to speedwork	1–2 x 5–10 km rest 5 km btwn
Long slow distance	Base/speed	Improves ability to do mileage builds training tolerance and improves recovery rate	Continuous
Active recovery	Base/speed	Assists recovery	Continuous
Spinning (cadence)			

90 MIN MOUNTAIN BIKE RACE

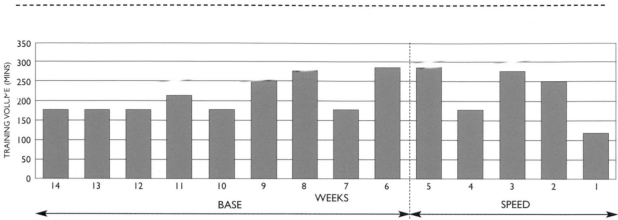

WEEK	14	13	12	11	10	9	8	7	6	5	4	3	2	1
SUBPHASE	1	1	2	2	2	2/3	2/3	2/3	4-6	4-6	4-6	6/7	6/7	6/7
FOCUS	Build	Recover	Build	Build	Recover	Build	Build	Recover	Build	Build	Recover	Build	Build	Recover
TOTAL TIME (MINS)	180	180	180	215	180	255	280	180	290	290	180	280	255	120
MON						D A Y	O F F							
TUES	40H	40E	40H	40H+Hbg	40E	60H+Hbg	60Fbg	40E	60RP+T	60RP+T	40E	60ST+A	60ST+A	40ST+A
WED						D A Y	O F F							
THURS	40E	40E	40E	60H	40E	60H	70H+Hbg	40E	80H+Hbg	80H+Hbg	40E	70H+Hbg	60H+Hbg	40E+C*
FRI						D A Y	O F F							
SAT	40E+BP	40E	40E+BP	40E+BP	40E	60A+BP	60A+BP	40E	60A+BP	60A+BP	40E	60RP+BP	60RP+BP	40E+C*
SUN	60E+T	60E+T	60E+T	75H+T	60E+T	75H+T	90H+T	60EC	90Fbg+C	90Fbg	60E+C	90Fbg+C	75E+C	EVENT

NOTES :

Suggested Practice Events: 90min Mountain Bike Race Simulation in weeks 7, 4 and 3

Speedwork: If club racing, remove speedwork. If you do wish to do speedwork, make sure that you use the correct intensities. Speedwork at the wrong intensity will not be beneficial for your training.

Off-road Training: Saturday and Sunday (Thursday is an optional extra off-road day)

Terrain: Practise mountain bike skills on the same terrain to measure your improvement

Transitions: During BP sessions, practise transitions on and off the bike over obstacles

KEY

	REPS	HR
BIKE		
E = EASY		LSD
T = TECHNIQUE		LSD
H = HILLS		
HBG = HILLS BIG GEAR	1 – 3 X 500M	
FBG = FLAT BIG GEAR	1 – 4 X 10 MIN	
RP = RACE PACE	1 – 2 X 5 MIN	AT
A = ACCELERATIONS	1 – 10 X 30S	UP TO AT
ST = STARTS	1 – 3 X 3 MIN	
C = COURSE OR SIMILAR CONDITIONS		LSD
BP = BIKE PUSH		LSD
	1 MIN RIDE,	
	1 MIN PUSH,	
	1 MIN CARRY	
C* = MUST RIDE COURSE	AND 1 MIN RUN	

2.5 HOUR MOUNTAIN BIKE RACE

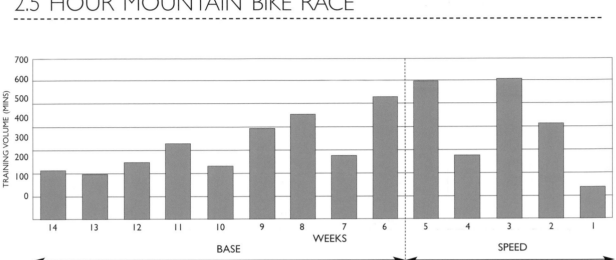

WEEK	14	13	12	11	10	9	8	7	6	5	4	3	2	1
SUBPHASE	1	1	2	2	2	2/3	2/3	2/3	4/5	4/5	4/5	6/7	6/7	6/7
MESOCYCLE	Build	Recover	Build	Build	Recover	Build	Build	Recover	Build	Build	Recover	Build	Build	Recover
TOTAL TIME (MINS)	220	200	250	330	230	395	460	280	540	600	280	610	415	140
MON														
TUES	40H	40E	60H	60H+Hbg	40E	75H+Hbg	75Fbg	60E	90RP	90RP	60E	90ST+A	75ST+A	60ST+A
WED	DAY OFF	DAY OFF	DAY OFF	60E+T	DAY OFF	60E+T	75E+T	DAY OFF	90E+T	90E+T	DAY OFF	90E+T	60E+T	DAY OFF
THURS	60E	60E	70E	80H	60E	80H	100H+Hbg	90E	120H+Hbg	120H+Hbg	60E	120H+Hbg	100H+Hbg	40E+C*
FRI	DAY OFF													
SAT	40E+BP	40E	40E+BP	40E+BP	40E	60A+BP	60A+BP	40E	60A+BP	60A+BP	40E	60RP+BP	60RP+BP	40E+C*
SUN	80E+T	60E+T	80E+T	100H	90E	120H	150H	90EC	180Fbg+C	240Fbg	120E+C	240Fbg+C	120E+C	EVENT

NOTES :

Suggested Practice Events: 2.5hr Mountain Bike Race Simulation in weeks 7, 4 and 3

Club Racing: Weekly club racing is recommended but use the suggested practice events as an opportunity to race more seriously

Speedwork: If club racing, remove speedwork. If you do wish to do speedwork, make sure that you use the correct intensities. Speedwork at the wrong intensity will not be beneficial for your training.

Off-road Training: Saturday and Sunday (Thursday is an optional extra off-road day)

KEY

BIKE	REPS	HR
E = EASY		LSD
T = TECHNIQUE		LSD
H = HILLS		
HBG = HILLS BIG GEAR	1 – 3 X 500M	
FBG = FLAT BIG GEAR	1 – 4 X 10 MIN	
RP = RACE PACE	1 – 2 X 5 MIN	AT
A = ACCELERATIONS	1 – 10 X 30S	UP TO AT
ST = STARTS	1 – 3 X 3 MIN	
C = COURSE OR SIMILAR CONDITIONS		LSD
BP = BIKE PUSH	1 MIN RIDE, 1 MIN PUSH, 1 MIN CARRY	
C* = MUST RIDE COURSE	AND 1 MIN RUN	

DISTANCE RUNNING TRAINING PROGRAMMES

19

Distance running covers races of varying lengths. The most common are 5 km, 10 km, Half Marathon and Marathon. The birth of marathon running is ascribed to the Athenian/ Persian battle of Marathon in 490BC, the story of which has become notoriously incorrect over the years.

The key things to remember are:

1. Start at the pace you can finish at. Most people start faster than they can finish. The key is to go for a negative or even split, running the second half of the event at an equal pace, or even quicker than the first.
2. Strength endurance is as crucial as distance training. This means doing hill efforts as part of your training.
3. The final third of the event is the hardest. You will use the same effort to run the final third as you need for the first two-thirds put together. It is more important to visualise this marker than to think about the halfway point.

4. Never run the advertised distance. An event is measured down the centre of the route. If you cut all the corners you will take some distance off the run, saving you time and energy.
5. Learn about running technique. This includes balance, foot strike and foot pick-up. Balance involves distributing your upper body weight equally on your pelvis. Your foot must strike the ground directly under your body so there is no loss of momentum. If your foot strikes the ground in front of your body there is a momentary loss of power which will slow you down at every step, like a brake. The difference per step is minimal, but in a marathon where you will be making 42, 000 steps you will notice the difference!
6. Stride Rate. Try to keep your stride rate even throughout the event. This will mean shortening your stride on the uphill sections to maintain rate.

Sport-specific training used for distance running

Type (intensity)	When initiated	Effect	Example
Power	—	—	—
Intensive sprints	—	—	—
Extensive sprints	Speed phase	Ability to employ race strategy, Leg speed	2–3 x 1–3 min rest to recovery
Submaximal	Speed phase	Improves max steady state race pace	4–6 x 6–8 min 4–1 min rest btwn or 20–30 min TT
Up-tempo	Late base, early speed	Transition from base to speedwork	1–2 x 5–10 km rest 5 km btwn
Long slow distance	Base/speed	Improves ability to do mileage, builds training tolerance and improves recovery rate	Continuous
Active recovery	Base/speed	Assists recovery	Continuous

10KM RUN

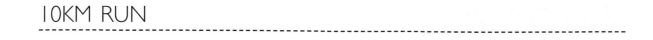

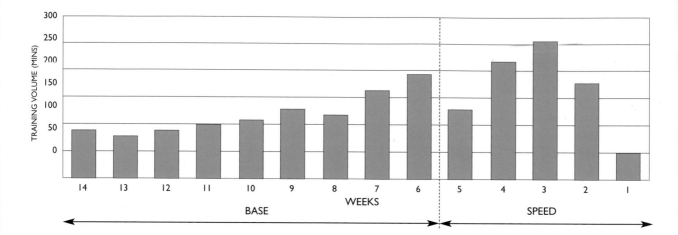

BASE   WEEKS   SPEED

WEEK	14	13	12	11	10	9	8	7	6	5	4	3	2	1
SUBPHASE	1/2	1/2	1/2	2/3	2/3	2/3	2/3	4	4	4	5/6	5/6	5/6	5/6
MESOCYCLE	Build	Build	Recover	Build	Build	Build	Recover	Build	Build	Recover	Build	Build	Recover	Recover
TOTAL TIME (MINS)	90	80	90	100	110	130	120	165	195	130	220	255	180	55
MON	DAY OFF													
TUES	20E	20E	20E	20A	20A	20A	20E	20A	20A	20E	30RP	30RP	20RP	20RP
WED	DAY OFF													
THURS	20E+T	20E+T	20E+T	20H	20H	30H	20E	40H+He	50H+He	30E	50H+He	60H+He	40H+He	30E
FRI	DAY OFF													
SAT	20E	20E	20E	20E	30E	30E	20E	30E	35E	30E	40S	45S	30S	5E
SUN	30E	20E	30E	40E	50E	60E	40C	70H	80H	60E	90C	90C	60C	EVENT

NOTES :

Suggested Practice Events: 5km Run in weeks 8, 5 and 3

KEY		REPS	HR
RUN			
E = EASY			LSD
T = TECHNIQUE			LSD
H = HILLS			
HE = HILLS EFFORTS		1 – 6 X 200M	
RP = RACE PACE		1 – 6 X 3 MIN	AT
UT = UP TEMPO		1 – 4 X 5 MIN	UT
A = ACCELERATIONS		1 – 10 X 30S	UP TO AT
C = COURSE OR SIMILAR CONDITIONS			LSD
S = HALF MARATHON RACE PACE			UT

ADVANCED 10KM RUN

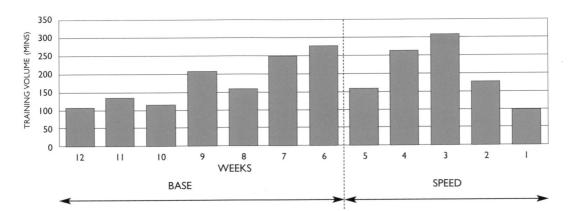

WEEK	12	11	10	9	8	7	6	5	4	3	2	1
SUBPHASE	2	2	1	3	3	4	4	4	5/6	5/6	5/6	5/6
MESOCYCLE	Build	Build	Recover	Build	Recover	Build	Build	Recover	Build	Build	Recover	Recover
EFFORT	RELAX								DILIGENT		FOCUS	
TOTAL TIME (MINS)	110	140	120	210	160	250	280	160	270	310	180	100
MON	DAY OFF			20E	DAY OFF	30E	30E	20E	30E	30E	20E	20E
TUES	20E	20H	20E	20H	30RP (2 x 200m)	40RP (2 x 400m)	40RP (2 x 600m)	30RP (4 x 400m)	40RP (4 x 600m)	40RP (4 x 800m)	30RP (4 x 400m)	30RP (3 x 200m)
WED	20E	20E	DAY OFF	30E	DAY OFF	40E	40E	DAY OFF	30E	40E	DAY OFF	
THURS	20H	30H (2 x 200m)	30E (2 x 200m)	30H+He (2 x 200m)	40H+He (2 x 200m)	40H+He (4 x 200m)	50H+He (2 x 500m)	30H+He (2 x 200m)	50H+He (4 x 500m)	60H + He (2 x 500m)	40H+He (3 x 200m)	30E
FRI	DAY OFF											
SAT	20H	30RP (2 x 400m)	30RP (2 x 400m)	40RP (3 x 600m)	30RP (4 x 600m)	30RP (4 x 800m)	40RP (4 x 800m)	20RP (2 x 200m)	30RP (4 x 1000m)	40RP (6 x 1000m)	30RP (4 x 400m)	20E
SUN	30H/C	40H/C	40H/C	50H/C	60H/C	70H/C	80H/C	60TT	90H/C	100C	60H/C	EVENT

NOTES :

Speedwork: Figures in brackets show speedwork required. If you know your
$^1/_2$ marathon time (or an estimate), calculate your interval times in this way:

1. Time to complete in mins (1.5 hr x 60 = 90 min) divided by the distance in km (21) e.g. 90 min divided by 21 = 4.29 min/km (speed)

2. Divide the distance of the interval by 1000 and multiply by the speed e.g. 200m divided by 1000 = 0.2 multiplied by 4.29 = 0.858 min

3. Multiply the decimal fraction of your result to work out the seconds e.g. 0.858 multiplied by 60 = 51.48 seconds

4. Run your interval in as close to 51 seconds as possible

Hill Efforts: Hill Efforts will strengthen your legs. Warm up on hills first, then find a hill with a shallow gradient and overall length of 200-500m. Run at marathon race pace, maintaining form and speed until you begin to lose breath. Relax, jog back down and recover before the next interval. Start with 1 rep at first and then build up to 6.

KEY		
	REPS	HR
RUN		
E = EASY		LSD
T = TECHNIQUE		LSD
H = HILLS		
HE = HILLS EFFORTS	1 – 6 X 200M	
RP = RACE PACE	1 – 3 X 4 MIN	AT
A = ACCELERATIONS	1 – 10 X 30S	UP TO AT
TT = TIME TRIAL		AT
C = COURSE OR SIMILAR CONDITIONS		

RECREATIONAL HALF MARATHON

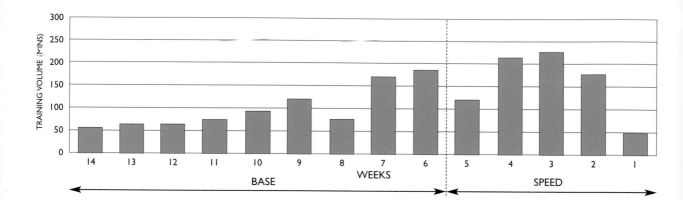

WEEK	14	13	12	11	10	9	8	7	6	5	4	3	2	1
SUBPHASE	1/2	1/2	1/2	2/3	2/3	2/3	2/3	4	4	4	5/6	5/6	5/6	5/6
MESOCYCLE	Build	Build	Recover	Build	Build	Build	Recover	Build	Build	Recover	Build	Build	Recover	Recover
TOTAL TIME (MINS)	60	70	70	80	100	130	80	180	200	130	230	240	190	50
MON	D A Y O F F													
TUES	20E	20E	20E	20H	20H	30H	20E	30H	30UT	30E	40UT	40UT	30UT	20E
WED	D A Y O F F													
THURS	20E+T	20E+T	20E+T	20E+T	30E+T	40H	20E	50H+He	60H+He	20E	60H+He	50TT	40E	20H
FRI	D A Y O F F													
SAT	D A Y O F F							30E	30E	30E	30S	30S	30S	10E
SUN	20E	30E	30C	40H	50H	60H	40C	70H	80H	60E	100C	120C	90C	EVENT

NOTES :

Suggested Practice Events: 5km Run in weeks 8 and 3

10km Run in week 5

KEY		
	REPS	**HR**
RUN		
E = EASY		LSD
T = TECHNIQUE		
H = HILLS		
HE = HILLS EFFORTS	1 – 6 X 200M	
UT = UP TEMPO	1 – 4 X 5 MIN	UT
S = SPEED	1 – 4 X 1 MIN	AT
A = ACCELERATIONS	1 – 10 X 30S	UP TO AT
TT = TIME TRIAL		UT
C = COURSE OR SIMILAR CONDITIONS		LSD

SEMI COMPETITIVE HALF MARATHON

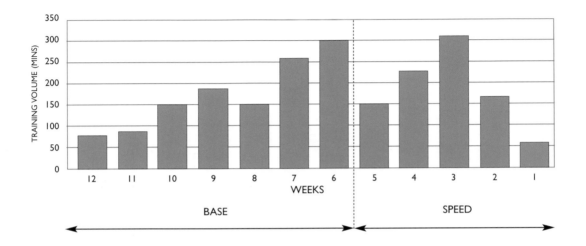

WEEK	12	11	10	9	8	7	6	5	4	3	2	1
SUBPHASE	1	1	2	2	2	2/3	2/3	2/3	4-6	4-6	4-6	4-6
MESOCYCLE	Build	Recover	Build	Build	Recover	Build	Build	Recover	Build	Build	Recover	Recover
EFFORT	RELAX		DILIGENT		RELAX	DILIGENT		RELAX		FOCUS		
TOTAL TIME (MINS)	80	90	150	190	150	260	300	150	230	310	170	60
MON	DAY OFF											
TUES	20H	20E	30H	30H + He	20E	40UT	50UT	30E	30E	50UT	30UT	30E
WED	DAY OFF		20E	20E	DAY OFF	30E	30E	DAY OFF	20E	30E	DAY OFF	
THURS	30E	30E	40E	40H	50E	60H + He	70H + He	30E	60H	80H + He	40H	20E
FRI	DAY OFF											
SAT	DAY OFF		20C	20C	20E	30C	30S	30E	20S	30S	20S	10E
SUN	30E	40C	60H	80H	60TT	100H	120H	60TT	100H	120C	80C	EVENT

NOTES :

Rest Weeks: You should have 3 complete rest weeks before starting this training programme

KEY		
	REPS	**HR**
RUN		
E = EASY		LSD
T = TECHNIQUE		LSD
H = HILLS		
HE = HILLS EFFORTS	1 – 6 X 200M	
UT = UP TEMPO	1 – 4 X 5 MIN	UT
S = SPEED	1 – 4 X 1 MIN	AT
A = ACCELERATIONS	1 – 10 X 30S	UP TO AT
TT = TIME TRIAL		UT
C = COURSE OR SIMILAR CONDITIONS		LSD

ADVANCED HALF MARATHON

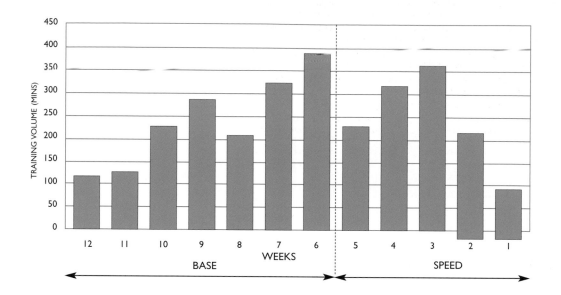

WEEK	12	11	10	9	8	7	6	5	4	3	2	1
SUBPHASE	1+2	1+2	2+3	2+3	2+3	2–4	2–4	2–4	5+6	5+6	5+6	5+6
MESOCYCLE	Build	Recover	Build	Build	Recover	Build	Build	Recover	Build	Build	Recover	Recover
EFFORT	RELAX		DILIGENT		RELAX	DILIGENT		RELAX		FOCUS		
TOTAL TIME (MINS)	120	130	230	290	210	330	400	230	320	370	240	110
MON	DAY OFF		20E	20E	20E	30E	40E	30E	40E	40E	30E	30E
TUES	20H (4 x 200m)	20RP (2 x 200m)	40RP (3 x 400m)	50RP (3 x 400m)	30RP (3 x 200m)	50RP (4 x 400m)	60RP (4 x 600m)	40RP (4 x 400m)	60RP (4 x 800m)	40RP (4 x 800m)	30RP (4 x 400m)	30RP (3 x 200m)
WED	20E	20E	30E	30E	30E	40E	40E	DAY OFF	30E	40E	30E	DAY OFF
THURS		30H+He (2 x 200m)	40H +He (3 x 200m)	50H+He (4 x 200m)	40H +He (2 x 200m)	70H+He (6 x 200m)	80H+He (4 x 500m)	40H+He (2 x 200m)	60H+He (4 x 500m)	90H+He (2 x 500m)	40H+He (3 x 200m)	30E
FRI	DAY OFF											
SAT	20RP (2 x 400m)	20RP (1 x 400m)	40RP (2 x 400m)	60RP (3 x 600m)	30RP (3 x 400m)	40RP (3 x 800m)	60RP (4 x 800m)	40RP (2 x 200m)	30RP (4 x 1000m)	40RP (6 x 1000m)	30RP (4 x 400m)	20E
SUN	30H/C	40H/C	60H/C	80H/C	60TT	100H/C	120H/C	80TT	100H/C	120C	80H/C	EVENT

NOTES :

Rest Weeks: You should have 3 complete rest weeks before starting this training programme

Speedwork: Figures in brackets show speedwork required. If you know your 1/2 marathon time (or an estimate), calculate your interval times in this way:

1. Time to complete in mins (1.5 hr x 60 = 90 min) divided by the distance in km (21) e.g. 90 min divided by 21 = 4.29 min/km (speed)

2. Divide the distance of the interval by 1000 and multiply by the speed e.g. 200m divided by 1000 = 0.2 multiplied by 4.29 = 0.858 min

3. Multiply the decimal fraction of your result to work out the seconds e.g. 0.858 multiplied by 60 = 51.48 seconds

4. Run your interval in as close to 51 seconds as possible

Hill Efforts: Hill Efforts will strengthen your legs. Warm up on hills first, then find a hill with a shallow gradient and overall length of 200-500m. Run at marathon race pace, maintaining form and speed until you begin to lose breath. Relax, jog back down and recover before the next interval. Start with 1 rep at first and then build up to 6.

KEY

RUN	REPS	HR
E = EASY		LSD
T = TECHNIQUE		LSD
H = HILLS		
HE = HILLS EFFORTS	1 – 6 X 200M	
UT = UP TEMPO	1 – 4 X 5 MIN	UT
RP = RACE PACE	1 – 4 X 30S	UT
A = ACCELERATIONS	1 – 10 X 30S	UP TO AT
TT = TIME TRIAL		UT
C = COURSE OR SIMILAR CONDITIONS		

RECREATIONAL MARATHON

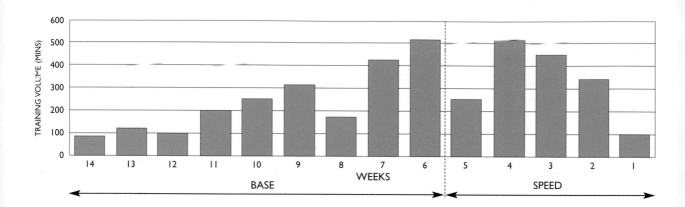

WEEK	14	13	12	11	10	9	8	7	6	5	4	3	2	1
SUBPHASE	1+2	1+2	1+2	2+3	2+3	2+3	2+3	2–4	2–4	2–4	5+6	5+6	5+6	5+6
MESOCYCLE	Build	Build	Recover	Build	Build	Build	Recover	Build	Build	Recover	Build	Build	Recover	Recover
TOTAL TIME (MINS)	90	120	90	190	250	310	170	425	510	250	510	445	340	100
MON	DAY OFF													
TUES	20E	30E	20E	40E	50H	60H	40E	75H	90UT	40E	90UT	75UT	60UT	40UT
WED	DAY OFF							40A	60A	DAY OFF	60A	60A	40A	20E
THURS	30E+T	30E+T	30E+T	40E+T	60H	80H	40E	100H	120H	90E	120H+He	100TTC	80H+He	30E+C
FRI	DAY OFF													
SAT	DAY OFF			30E	40E	50H+He	30E	60H+He	60H+He	30E	60S	60S	40S	10E+C
SUN	40E	60E	40C	80H	100H	120H	60C	150H	180C	90E	180H	150C	120C	EVENT

NOTES :

Suggested Practice Events: 10km Run in weeks 8 and 3
21km Run in week 5

KEY		
	REPS	HR
RUN		
E = EASY		LSD
T = TECHNIQUE		LSD
H = HILLS		
HE = HILLS EFFORTS	1 – 6 X 200M	
UT = UP TEMPO	1 – 4 X 5 MIN	UT
S = SPEED	1 – 4 X 1 MIN	AT
A = ACCELERATIONS	1 – 10 X 30S	UP TO AT
TT = TIME TRIAL		UT
C = COURSE OR SIMILAR CONDITIONS		LSD

STANDARD MARATHON

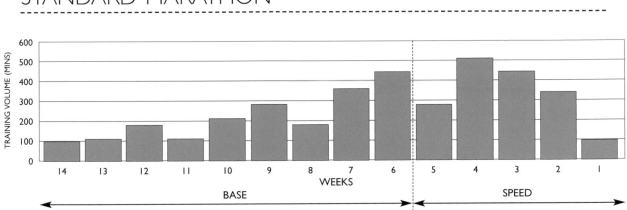

WEEK	14	13	12	11	10	9	8	7	6	5	4	3	2	1
SUBPHASE	1	1	1+2	2+3	2+3	2+3	2+3	2–4	2–4	2–4	5+6	5+6	5+6	5+6
MESOCYCLE	Build	Recover	Build	Recover	Build	Build	Recover	Build	Build	Recover	Build	Build	Recover	Recover
TOTAL TIME (MINS)	100	110	180	110	210	285	180	360	445	280	510	445	340	100
MON	DAY OFF													
TUES	20E	20E	30E	20E	30E	45H	30E	60H	75UT	40E	90UT	75UT	60UT	40UT
WED	DAY OFF		20E	DAY OFF	30E	40E	DAY OFF	50A	60A	DAY OFF	60A	60A	40A	20E
THURS	30E	30E	40H	30E	40E	60H	40E	80H	100H	80E	120H	100TT/C	80H	30E
FRI	DAY OFF													
SAT	20E	20E	30F	20E	30E	40E	30E	50E	60H	40E	60S	60S	40S	10E
SUN	30E	40E	60E	40H	80H	100H	80C	120H	150C	120E	180H	150C	120C	EVENT

NOTES :

Time Trial: Run 15 km at marathon race pace, no faster.

KEY		
	REPS	**HR**
RUN		
E = EASY		LSD
T = TECHNIQUE		LSD
H = HILLS		
HE = HILLS EFFORTS	1 – 6 X 200M	
UT = UP TEMPO	1 – 4 X 5 MIN	UT
S = SPEED	1 – 4 X 1 MIN	AT
A = ACCELERATIONS	1 – 10 X 30S	UP TO AT
TT = TIME TRIAL 15 KM		UT
C = COURSE OR SIMILAR CONDITIONS		LSD

ADVANCED MARATHON

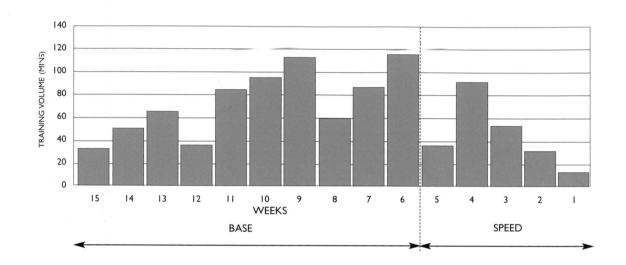

NOTES :

Please refer to the Detailed Training Programme Keys for more information.

KEY

FS = FOOT STRIKE
LT = LEG TURNOVER
F = RUNNING FLUIDITY/RELAXED
SH = RELAXED SHOULDERS
BR = RELAXED BREATHING
PO = PUSH OFF
AS = ARM SWING
PU = PICK UPS
UP = UP RIGHT
NUT = EVENT NUTRITION
EFT = EVEN EFFORT
CRS = RUNNING GOOD LINES
RHM = RHYTHM

	15	14	13	12	11	10	9	8	7	6	5	4	3	2	1
WEEK	15	14	13	12	11	10	9	8	7	6	5	4	3	2	1
SUBPHASE	1+2	1+2	1+2	1+2	2+3	2+3	2+3	2+3	2–4	2–4	2–4	5+6	5+6	5+6	5+6
MESOCYCLE	BUILD	BUILD	BUILD	RECOVER	BUILD	BUILD	BUILD	RECOVER	BUILD	BUILD	RECOVER	BUILD	BUILD	RECOVER	RECOVER
TOTAL	34	52	66	38	86	98	115	62	89	117	38	94	54	32	14
MON															
ES															
AT															
UT															
ACC															
He															
LC															
TERR															
TECH															
TACTIC															
TUES	6	8	10	6	16	18	22	16	8	20	8	16	8	6	4
ES											5KM RACE	5KM RACE		5KM RACE	
AT												TEMPO	TEMPO		TEMPO
UT										6 X 1000		6 X 400			3 X 400
ACC															
He	2	4	6		6	8	10	3	10	4					
LC															
TERR	RH	H	H	RH	RH	H	H	RH	H	H	F	F	F	F	F
TECH	F/SH	BR/RHM	F/SH	BR/RHM	F/SH	BR/RHM	F/SH	F/SH	F/SH	BR/RHM	F/SH	BR/RHM	F/SH	BR/RHM	F/SH
TACTIC	RHM	CRS	RHM	CRS	RHM	CRS	RHM	CRS	RHM	RHM	CRS	RHM	CRS	RHM	CRS
WED	4	6	8		10	12	12		10	12		8	6		
ES															
AT															
UT															
ACC	2	2	4		4	6			4	6		8	6		
He															
LC															
TERR	F	F	F		F	F			F	F		F	F		
TECH															
TACTIC															
THURS	10	12	14	6	16	20	25	10	12	25	6	20	12	6	6
ES															
AT															
UT															
ACC															
He	4	6	8	2	10	12	16	6	8	20	6	12	8	2	2
LC		1	2		2	2			1	2		2			
TERR	H	HH	HH	RH	HH	HH	RH	RH	H	H	RH	H	H	RH	RH
TECH	LT/PU	PO/AS	LT/PU	PO/AS	LT/PU	PO/AS	LT/PU	LT/PU	PO/AS	LT/PU	PO/AS	LT/PU	PO/AS	LT/PU	PO/AS
TACTIC	CRS	CRS	NUT/EFT	CRS	CRS	NUT/EFT	CRS	CRS	CRS	NUT/EFT	CRS	NUT/EFT	CRS	CRS	CRS
FRI		6	8		8	8	10		8	10		8			
ES															
AT															
UT															
ACC															
He															
LC															
TERR		F	F		F	F			F	F		F			
TECH															
TACTIC															
SAT	6	8	10	6	12	14	16	4	16	12	8	12	8	6	4
ES															
AT															
UT		4 X 400	6 X 400		2 X 1000	3 X 1000	4 X 1000	2 X 200	4 X 1000	8 X 1000		6 X 1000		4 X 400	4 X 200
ACC		3% INCLINE	3% INCLINE		3% INCLINE	3% INCLINE	3% INCLINE								
He															
LC															
TERR	H	H	H	F	H	H	F		H	H	F	RH	RH	F	F
TECH	F/SH	BR/RHM	F/SH	RHM	BR/RHM	F/SH	RHM		F/SH	BR/RHM	F/SH	BR/RHM	F/SH	BR/RHM	RHM
TACTIC	RHM	CRS	RHM	CRS	CRS	RHM	CRS		CRS	RHM	CRS	RHM	CRS	RHM	CRS
SUN	8	12	16	20	24	26	30	32	35	38	16	30	20	14	MARA
ES								TT							
AT								ON	ON	ON		ON	ON	ON	
UT								COURSE	COURSE	COURSE		COURSE	COURSE	COURSE	
ACC															
He															
LC															
TERR	H	H	HH	RH	HH	HH	HH				RH				
TECH	FS/LT	FS/LT	FS/LT	FS/LT	FS/LT	FS/LT	FS/LT	FS/LT	FS/LT	FS/LT	FS/LT	FS/LT	FS/LT	FS/LT	
TACTIC	CRS	NUT/EFT	CRS	CRS	NUT/EFT	CRS	CRS	CRS	CRS	NUT/EFT	CRS	NUT/EFT	CRS	NUT/EFT	

Key (right-hand columns, repeated for each day):

	REPS	HEART RATE
ES		
AT	REPS X 50M	N/A
UT	REPS X DIST	AT
ACC	REPS X DIST	UT
He	REPS X 30SECS	UP TO AT
LC	REPS X 200/500M	N/A
TERR	REPS X 10MINS	N/A
TECH	N/A	
TACTIC	N/A	

APPENDIX 1: USEFUL CALCULATIONS

To calculate speed and average speed

For minutes per kilometre (min/km)

time to complete workout (min) ÷ distance covered in workout (km) = speed (min/km)

e.g. 30 min ÷ 6 km = 5 min/km

For kilometres per hour (kph)

distance (km) covered in workout ÷ time (min) to complete work out x 60 = speed (kph)

e.g. 39 km ÷ 80 min x 60 = 29.3 km

To calculate duration

Using min/km

distance (km) x speed (min/km) = duration (min)

e.g. 6 km x 5 min/km = 30 min

Using kph

distance (km) ÷ speed (kph) x 60 = duration (min)

e.g. 39 km ÷ 29.3 kph x 60 = 80 min

Using m/sec

Either:
distance (m) ÷ speed (m/sec) = duration (sec)

e.g. 500 m ÷ 1.18 m/sec = 425 sec

Or:
distance (m) ÷ speed (m/sec) ÷ 60 = duration (min)

e.g. 2000 m ÷ 4.76 ÷ 60 = 7 min

To calculate distance

Using min/km

time (min) ÷ speed (min/km) = distance (km)

e.g. 30 min ÷ 5 min/km = 6 km

Using kph

time (min) x speed (kph) ÷ 60 = distance (km)

e.g. 80 min x 29.3 kph ÷ 60 = 39 km

Using m/sec

> Either:
> time (sec) × speed (m/sec) = distance (m)
>
> e.g. 425 sec × 1.18 m/sec = 500 m
>
> or:
> time (min) × speed (m/sec) × 60 = distance (m)
>
> e.g. 7 min × 4.76 m/sec × 60 = 2000 m

To calculate average weight, resting pulse, hours sleep, training time/distance

Total up each of the variable from each day during the week you are in, then divide by the number of days in the week. For weight, resting pulse and sleep, this will always be seven days if you are filling the log book out correctly. For training, divide by the number of days/workouts.

For example, for distance:
10 km + 16 km + 10 km + 20 km + 10 km + 30 km = 96 km
Divide by 6 for 6 workouts: 96 km ÷ 6 workouts = 16 km average

To calculate percentage increase/decrease

From total training time/distance and last week's total calculate percentage increase/decrease in training volume.

> total training time/distance for week (min/km) ÷ last week's total (min/km) × 100 − 100 = percentage increase or decrease
>
> e.g. Total training this week = 96 km
>   Total training last week = 87 km
>
> 96 km ÷ 87 km × 100 − 100 = 10.3% (increase)
> 87 km ÷ 96 km × 100 − 100 = −9.4% (decrease)

To calculate percentage field

> placing in race ÷ total number of competitors × 100 = % field
>
> e.g. 10th placing ÷ 750 competitors × 100 = 1.3%
> (You came in the top 1.3% of the field)

To calculate percentage time difference

> your time for race (min or sec) ÷ 1st-place-getter's time (min or sec) × 100 − 100 = % time difference
>
> e.g. 75 min ÷ 62 min × 100 − 100 = 21%
> (You took 21% longer to complete the race)

BIBLIOGRAPHY

Armstrong, Lance and Carmichael, Chris. *The Lance Armstrong Performance Program*, Rodale, 2006

Ashcroft, Frances *Life at Extremes, The Science of Survival*, Flamingo/Harper Collins, 2001

Brooks, G. A. and Fahey, D. F. *Fundamentals of Human Performance*, Macmillan Publishing, 1984**

Brotherhood, J. R. 'Nutrition and Sports Performance', *Sports Medicine*, 1984*

Burke, Edmund (ed.). *Precision Heart Rate Training*, Human Kinetics, 1998

Burke, E. R. *Science of Cycling*, Human Kinetics, 1986**

Burke, E. R. *Medical and Scientific Aspects of Cycling*, Human Kinetics**

Burke, L. and Read, R. 'Sports Nutrition, Approaching the Nineties', *Sports Medicain*, 1989

Burlingame et al. *The Concise NZ Food Composition Tables*, NZ Institute for Crop and Food Research Ltd, 1993

Coleman, E. *Eating for Endurance*, Bull Publishing Co., 1988*

Edwards, S. *The Heart Rate Monitor Book*, Fleet Feet Press, 1992*

Finch, Michael. *Triathlon Training*, Human Kinetics, 2004

Food for Health, Report of the Nutrition Taskforce, New Zealand Department of Health, New Zealand, 1991

Foods, Nutrition and Sports Performance, Statement from International Conference, Feb, 1991

Friel, Joe. *The Cyclists Training Bible*, Velopress, 1996

Friel, Joe. *The Triathletes Training Bible*, Velopress, 1998

Friel, Joe and Bryn, Gordon. *Going Long*, Velopress, 2003

Gisolfi, C. and Duchman, S. 'Guidelines for Optimal Replacement Beverages for Different Athletic Events', *Medicine & Science in Sports and Exercise*, Vol. 24, No. 6, 1992

Hahn, A. G. *State of the Art Review, no. 31: The Physiological Rationale for Altitude Training*, National Sports Research Centre, Australian Sports Commission, 1992

Haymes, E. M. and Wells, C. L. *Environment and Human Performance*, Human Kinetics 1986

Hawley, John and Burke, Louise. *Peak Performance*, Allen & Unwin, 1998

Hellemans, I. 'Nutritional Considerations for Physically Active Adults and Athletes in New Zealand', New Zealand Dietetic Association Position Paper, Nov, 1991

Hellemans, J. Triathlon: *A Complete Guide to Training and Racing*, Reed Publishing, 1993*

Hinault, B. and Genzling, C. Road Racing: Technique and Racing, Reed Publishing, 1993*

Howley, E. T. and Franks, B. D. Health Fitness Instructors Handbook, second edition, Human Kinetics, 1992**

Inge, K. and Brukner, P. Food for Sport, William Heineman, 1986*

Janssen, Peter. *Lactate Threshold Training*, Human Kinetics, 2001

Janssen, P. G. J. M. Training Lactate Pulse Rate, Polar Electro Oy Publishers, 1987**

Lemond, G. and Gordis, K. *Greg Lemond's Complete Book of Bicycling*, The Putnam Publishing Group, 1990*

Longhurst, K. and Blundell, N. *State of the Art Review, no. 9: Anaerobic Threshold and Endurance Performance*, National Sports Research Centre, Australian Sports Commission, 1986

MacKinnon, L. T. and Hooper, S. *State of the Art Review, no. 26: Overtraining, National Sports Research Centre*, Australian Sports Commission, 1991

MacKinnon, L. and Hooper, S. *Training Logs: An Effective Method of Monitoring Overtraining and Tapering – Coaches' Report*, National Sports Research Centre, Australian Sprts Commission, 1991

Maffetone, P. and Mantell, M. E. *The High Performance Heart*, Bicycle Books Inc. 1991*

McArdle, W. D. Katch, F. I. and Katch, V. L. Exercise *Physiology*, Led & Febiger, 1986**

Morris, David. *Performance Cycling*, Ragged Mountain Press, 2003

Pearce, J. *Eat to Compete*, Heinemann Reed, Auckland, 1990*

Sharkey, B. J. *Physiology of Fitness*, third edition, Human Kinetics, 1990**

Sleamaker, R. *Serious Training for Serious Athletes*, Leisure Press*

Sports Nutrition, Sports & Cardiovascular Nutritionists (SCAN), The American Dietetic Association, 1988

Wilbur, Randall, L. *Altitude Training and Athletic Performance*, Human Kinetics, 2004

Wootton, S, Nutrition for Sport, Simon & Schuster Ltd, 1989*

RECOMMENDED READING

Adventure Racing by Jacques Marais and Lisa de Speville (Human Kinetics, Illinois USA, 2004)

Adventure Racing, the Ultimate Guide by Liz Caldwell and Barry Siff, (Velopress, Colorado USA, 2001)

Bike Racing 101 by Kendra Wenzel and Rene Wenzel (Human Kinetics, Illinois USA, 2003)

Fixing your Feet by John Vonhof (Wilderness Press, California, 1997)

Food for Fitness (3rd edition) by Anita Bean (A & C Black, London, 2006)

Maximum Performance for Cyclists by Michael J. Ross (Velopress, Colorado USA, 2005)

Performing in Extreme Environments by Lawrence E. Armstrong (Human Kinetics, Illinois USA, 2000)

Racing Tactics for Cyclists by Thomas Prehn (Velopress, Colorado USA, 2004)

Road Racing, Technique & Training by Bernard Hinault and Claude Genzling (Vitesse Press, Vermont USA, 1988)

Runners World Guide to Adventure Racing by Ian Adamson (Rodale, New York, USA, 2004)

Serious Mountain Biking by Ann Trombley (Human Kinetics, Illinois USA, 2005)

Slaying the Dragon by Michael Johnson (Hodder & Stoughton, London, 1996)

Sports Speed by George Dintiman, Bob Ward and Tom Tellez (Human Kinetics, Illinois USA, 1997)

Sports Training Principles (5th edition) by Frank W. Dick O.B.E. (A & C Black, London, 2007)

Survival of the Fittest by Mike Stroud (Vintage, London, 1999)

The Complete Fliers Handbook by Brian Clegg (Pan, London, 2002)

The Complete Guide to Adventure Racing by Don Mann and Kara Schaad (Hatherleigh Press, New York USA, 2001)

The Complete Guide to Sports Nutrition by Anita Bean (A & C Black, London, 2006)

The Complete Guide to Stretching (3rd edition) by Christopher M. Norris (A & C Black, London, 2007)

Training and Racing with a Power Meter by Hunter Allen and Andrew Coggan (Velopress, Colorado USA, 2006)

Travel Fitness by Johnson, R., and Tulin, W., (Human Kinetics, Illinois USA, 1995)

Also by the Author:

Precision Training (Reed Publishing, New Zealand, 1998)

Spinning-Cycling Workouts for the Road & Stationary Trainers (Reed Publishing, New Zealand. 1998)

Personal Best (Reed Publishing, New Zealand, 2000)

Half Marathon (Random House, London, 2006)

Ironman Pack (Performance Lab, New Zealand, 2006)

INDEX

Page numbers with 't' show tables. Figures are shown in italics.

active recovery (AR) 20–1, 28, 41–2, 67, 127
aerobic threshold 77, 117
altitude training 180–8
anaerobic threshold (AT) 35, 37, 57, 113–18, 127
    see also submaximal intensity (SM) training
attack 171–3
attitude 6, 17, 170, 173–6

base phase 6–7, 16–17, 69, 70, 80, 99
    and races 84–5
    and subphases 48, 49–55
    see also individual sports
blueprints 133–42, 163

coaches 6, 175, 177–9
cold, training in 191–2
Conconi test 114–18
cycles in training 21–6
cycling 21–2, 86, 161t
    base phase *50*, 51, 53, 54–5, 61–3, 80
    and heart rates 46–7
    mesocycles 92, 96t
    and overtraining 127
    peak mileage 72–3, 144t
    racing 86
    speed phase 56–63, 75t, 80t, 81t
    and strength testing 120
    and strength training 109

defense 173–6
dehydration *see* hydration
diminishing returns 31–2, 65
duathlon:
    base phase 23t, *50*, 51, 54, 55t
    peak mileage 72t, 149–50t
    racing 86
    speed phase 23t, *50*, 57t, 58t
duration 5, 8

energy systems 7–8, 192

fat 119, 195–6, 199t, 201, 202, 208
fitness testing 111–21
flexibility 3–4, 104, 118
    see also stretching
frequency of training 3, 6

goals 2, 4, 5, 10–13, 95, 132
grunt 33–4, 48

heart rate monitors 36, 40, 41, 77, 126, 186
    and time trials 45–7
heart rates 35–47, 49, 113, 116–18, 126–7
heat, training in189–91
high-intensity (HI) training 44, 75
hydration 28, 29, 172, 190, 197, 203–4, 206–7

illness 125, 128
in-season training 66, 70–1
injury 27, 30, 104, 128–9
intensities 5, 13, *14*, 34–45, 61, 76t
    and altitude training 182–3
    and heart rates 34–41
    and speed phase 78–81, 82–3
    and subphases 61
ironman 12, *62*, 70, 72t, 86, 148t

Karvonen formula 37, *38–9*
kayaking 52, 55, 72t, 162t

load subphases 52–4
load/speed subphases 54–6
log books 6, 133, 164–6
long slow distance (LSD) 42, 76t
low intensity (LO) training 41–2, 75, 127–8

maintenance 4, 30–4
medical problems 124–5, 128
mental attitude 6, 170, 173–6
mesocycles 24, *25–6*, 81–2, 96–7, 156–60
    see also individual sports
microcycles 21–3, 22–3t, 96, 134–41, 146–56t
mileage 71–3, 134–7, 161–2
minerals 201–3

mistakes 97–9, 103–4
monitors, heart rate 36, 40, 41, 77, 126, 186
mountain biking *see* cycling
multisport:
   and heart rates 47
   mileage 72t
   racing 86
   and speed phases 57t, 58t, 59t
   and strength testing 120
   and subphases *50*, 51t, 52t, 54t, 55t

nutrition 28, 102, 111, 172, 195–208

orthostatic heart rate test 37, *39*, 126
overcompensation 29–30, 31t, 93–4
overspeed 60–1
overtraining 27, 121–8

peak-mileage 71–3, 134–7, 143–56t
peaking 18, 19–20, 70–1, 90
percentage ranges 156–60t
performance 13, *14*, 21, *21*
periodisation 14, 67–70
planning 2–7, 11–13
power subphases 59–60, 75t, 76t
preparation 6–7, 51, 167–70
programmes 3, 6, 11–12, 132–63, 146–7t
progression 32–4, *49*
protein 200–1

race pace (RP) training 44–5
racing 9, 19, 40–1, 78, 83–90, 102
recovery 3, 24, 26–30
   active (AR) 20–1, 41–2, 42, 67, 127
   and overtraining 128
rowing:
   and base phases *50*, 51t, 52, 54–5
   and duration conversions 162t
   and heart rates 47
   and load subphases 53
   and microcycles 23t
   peak mileage 72t, 145t, 153t
   and racing 86
   and speed phase 57t, 58, 59t, 60t, 75t
   and strength testing 120
running 12
   and base phase 23t, *50*, 51t, 53, 54–5
   and heart rates 47
   and load 53

mesocycles 82t
   overtraining 127
   peak mileage 72t, 154–6t
   racing 86
   speed phases 56, 57t, 58, 59t, 75t, 77

seasons 14–21, 66–71, 133–4
speed phase 18, 48–9, 56–60, 74–83
   and mesocycles *25*, 156–60
   mistakes 97–8
   and periodisation 69
   testing 119
   see also individual sports
sprints 58–9, 75t, 76t, 78
strategies for improvement 65–6
strength 73–4, 106, 108–11, 119–20
stretching 100–2, 104–6, *107–8*
submaximal intensity (SM) training 35, 37, 38, 41, 43, 75, 76t
subphases 48, 49–64, 140
swimming 52, 53, 55, 93t, 109, 162t

tapering 18–19, 69, 86, 88–90, 99
technique 2, 4, 6, 20–1, 172–3
time 5–6, 7, 61, *62*, *63*, 69–70
   saving 10–11, 90–7
   see also periodisation
time trials 45–7, 77–8
tiredness 24, 100, 104
training cycles 21–6
training sessions 63–4
travel 192–4
triathlon:
   base phases *50*, 51t, 52t, 54t, 55t
   fitness testing 120
   peak mileage 72t, 146–7t
   racing 86
   speed phases 57t, 58t, 75t
   training 22t, 26t

up-tempo (UT) 42, 49, 76t, 80t

vitamins 210–11
VO$_2$max 111–14
volume 5, 13–14, *14*, 17, 182

warming up/down 4, 28, 100–3
working programmes 132–3, 163